Committed

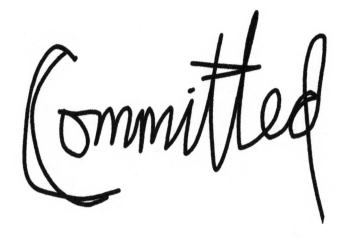

Committed

A Memoir of Madness

in the Family

PAOLINA MILANA

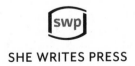

SHE WRITES PRESS

Copyright © 2021, Paolina Milana

All rights reserved. No part of this publication may be reproduced, distributed, or transmitted in any form or by any means, including photocopying, recording, digital scanning, or other electronic or mechanical methods, without the prior written permission of the publisher, except in the case of brief quotations embodied in critical reviews and certain other noncommercial uses permitted by copyright law. For permission requests, please address She Writes Press.

Published 2021
Printed in the United States of America
Print ISBN: 978-1-64742-042-0
E-ISBN: 978-1-64742-043-7
Library of Congress Control Number: 2020925791

For information, address:
She Writes Press
1569 Solano Ave #546
Berkeley, CA 94707

Interior design by Tabitha Lahr

She Writes Press is a division of SparkPoint Studio, LLC.
All company and/or product names may be trade names, logos, trademarks, and/or registered trademarks and are the property of their respective owners.

Included photographs are from the author's personal archive.

This book is dedicated to madness and to all of the people and circumstances in my life that have helped me find the magic within.

*"You're only given a little spark of madness.
You mustn't lose it."*
—ROBIN WILLIAMS

AUTHOR'S NOTE

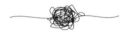

THE PEOPLE AND PLACES AND EVENTS depicted here are all real, as true to my memory as possible. In order to preserve anonymity, a few names and, in certain cases, identifying details have been changed. No composite characters or events were created in writing this book. Some people and events were purposely omitted, but that omission has no impact on the integrity of the story. It is my hope that the truth I share does justice to all those involved and that my story is read as one of faith, inspiration, commonalities, understanding, forgiveness, and resilience.

CONTENTS

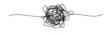

PROLOGUE

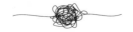

*"You've got to put the past behind you
before you can move on."*
—FORREST GUMP

THIS BOOK IS THE COMPANION to *The S Word*, my memoir about secrets. It took me a decade or so of therapy to process my childhood and then more than ten years to put pen to paper to tell it. The first part of my story published in 2015 and shared my memories of what it was like for me coming of age surrounded by crazy. From the age of about ten until I left home for college, I learned to keep secrets to survive: as a first-generation Sicilian Catholic "good girl" trying to serve as family caregiver; as the daughter of a mother who hid her paranoid schizophrenia from doctors and the outside world for far too long; and as a teenager exploring her own sexual awakening and finding herself in too deep with trusted authority figures who abused their power.

And I did survive.

Committed, this book you now hold in your hands, is the rest of this story. It shares my memories of being a college student trying to be "normal" while keeping my family cray-cray at bay. And it focuses not just on my mother's mental illness, which still raged on, but on that of my little sister, who at age twenty-four also was diagnosed with paranoid schizophrenia.

Insanity had taken root in my family tree, and I was tasked with tending our garden.

This part of my story is the end of what came before as much as it is the beginning of what would come as a result. By the time *Committed* publishes, it will be twenty years since I escaped the madness I was born into and journeyed further, learning to balance my own madness with the magic that also resided in me. The road has been long and, in truth, never-ending. But this book represents closure for me, and how I finally began to put the past behind me in order to move on.

Part One:
The Beginning of The End

"One's mind, once stretched by a new idea, never regains its original dimensions."
—Oliver Wendell Holmes, Sr.

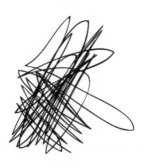

CHAPTER ONE: **COLLEGE**

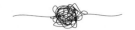

August 1985

ONE YEAR.

I took a deep breath and looked around at my windowless cell of a dorm room. Could I really survive living here?

When Iowa State University told me I had signed up too late for the Fall 1985 semester and would be placed in temporary housing, I never imagined *this* to be what they meant. I walked over to the army cot that was to serve as my bed and sat on it. Kicking off my sneakers, I absentmindedly nodded, now understanding fully that for ISU, the words "temporary housing" were synonymous with "kitchenette": my home away from home was the place where the other students would be washing their dishes and making use of shared cleaning supplies. I would be living in the very center room of the all-freshman, all-female sixth floor of a building called Willow that looked prison-like from the outside, and, according to the campus map, was the residence hall located the farthest from any of the classrooms.

What had I signed up for?

I could still see that look on my papà's face when he'd dropped me off just a few hours earlier and gotten a tour of where I'd be staying. His expression had clearly asked, *This is where you'd rather live than your own home?*

My silent response had been, *Yes*, without hesitation. But now, left here by myself, I was no longer sure.

I had chosen the cot to the right of the sink, the one farthest from the door that was the only way in or out. I could already imagine girls gabbing in the hallway right outside at all hours of the day and night, and I made a mental note to pick up some ear plugs. Maybe I'd get two sets and give one to my roommate, who had yet to show up.

As I turned to face the faded yellow walls, I became fascinated by their appearance: I couldn't tell if they were concrete or cinder blocks or real bricks. Maybe the walls weren't made of anything permanent. Maybe they were like the Hollywood movie sets constructed of Styrofoam. I reached over with my hand and started stroking the bumpy texture. Ouch! I pulled away and made another mental note: *No leaning against the very hard, very real, and very razor-sharp walls.*

I didn't know what else to do with myself, other than sit and think. And thinking wasn't always such a good thing. The voices in my head—when given the chance—had *a lot* of opinions, none of which were necessarily words of wisdom. I used my time to argue with them:

Why don't you unpack?

And put my stuff where?

Oh, right. Why don't you take a shower?

Where *are* the showers?

I looked down at what I was wearing: A pair of too-tight Gloria Vanderbilt jeans, so old and faded that they barely had any blue left in them, and a grayish-white cotton T-shirt with smudges of dirt left over from moving boxes. I lifted my arms up overhead to tighten the ponytail holder around my long, curly brown hair—which, surprisingly, wasn't as frizzy as usual. Chicago in August was hot enough. Ames, Iowa, was even hotter, with temperatures in the high 90s and humidity that made it feel well over 100 degrees.

Why don't you call home?

Are you kidding? I just travelled 360 miles to get away. Let me enjoy a little peace.

I wished the voices in my head would give it a rest. Or at least not ask such stupid questions. But I supposed I should be grateful. It wasn't as if they were talking to me the way Mamma's did, telling her that her own family meant her harm. Hers were symptoms of her paranoid schizophrenia. Mine were normal. I hoped.

What will she be like?

Who?

Your roomie.

I don't know. I hope she's like me: a third-year student and not a first-year.

You should have just stayed at UIC. What a mistake to have come here.

Two years as an undergrad at University of Illinois at Chicago taught me lots, including that it was too close to home. I needed out.

What do you think she's going to say about our living quarters? What if she wanted the cot you chose?

Why would it matter? There's really no difference.

Actually, there is. Your side has cabinets under the sink stocked with cleaning supplies, while her side has a tall closet where the vacuum and brooms are kept.

Seriously?

What if she's as prickly as the walls?

Look, I don't care what she is. She can be anything at all—except a J-O-C-K. It's bad enough I weigh a couple hundred pounds. I don't need some physical fitness nut sizing me up and judging everything I eat and all the exercise I don't do.

As if on cue, the door to the room swung open and in swaggered my roommate.

I was shocked into momentary silence as I took her in: Not much taller than the doorknob, she sported short, layered, sandy blond hair and wore grey sweat shorts, a grey sweatshirt that had the arms cut off so the edges were now frayed and white high-tops. A pair of white low-top sneakers hung by their shoestrings over her right shoulder. With her left hand, she lifted her ISU red and yellow duffel bag, showing off her seriously impressive and clearly defined biceps, and tossed it into the center of the room.

She nodded in my direction, then turned to pull a few more bags and boxes in from the hallway.

Frozen in place, I could only blink, which I did a few times, in disbelief. I felt as if I had to be starring in an episode of some hidden camera reality or prank-type television show. Pretty soon, someone would jump out from somewhere and say, "Smile, you're on *Candid Camera*." That had to be it. She was a J-O-C-K. Not the weekend warrior kind, the real deal. I could see it in how she looked and carried herself. She was the very thing I had hoped I would *not* get stuck with. What were the chances? It had to be staged.

When she finished hauling in her stuff, she shut the door and turned to look at me.

I unfroze and rose as quickly as I could from my cot. "Hi," I stammered out. "I'm Paolina." Extending my hand, I took a step forward, and we shook.

"Beth," she said in a voice much softer than I had expected.

After releasing my hand, Beth put her hands on her hips and scanned the room. Slowly, she nodded, a smirk spreading across her makeup-free, cherub-like face. "Wow." She chortled. "So this is it?"

Something about her laugh and her presence calmed me. The committee in my head chimed in. For once, we were in agreement: *We like her.*

So do I.

Besides, it's not really one full year; it's only nine months—August to May. You'll survive.

I nodded. Of course I would survive.

At the age of twenty, I felt as if I had twice as many years' worth of living already under my belt. But *this* was the year that would be like no other. I had enough money (correction: almost enough) to attend an away school for this *one* year. This was my year to be just about me, with no past to drag alongside me. No family to care for. No one here at ISU would know anything about my home or my history growing up, surrounded by madness. For the first time in my life, I would be just me. And I could be—would be—*normal*.

Or so I hoped.

I smiled back at Beth, "Yeah. This is it."

I SPENT THAT FIRST DAY of freedom from my family and the madness I had left back home exploring the ISU campus grounds. The Willow Residence Hall was located at the far southeast corner of campus, right next to the recreation fields at the busy intersection of Lincoln Way and North University Boulevard. The shortest path to my closest classes would require a half-mile hike each way, or so said the ISU campus map. I sweated at the very thought of it. Walking, or any type of activity, really wasn't my thing, especially in the sweltering August heat. Not that I was a big fan of the cold; I refused to even think of what it would be like during the dead of winter. I shut my eyes momentarily, turned my face upward toward the sunshine, and let the beads of sweat trickle down the sides of my face.

So this is what it was like to be normal: just me walking by myself, trying to find my own way . . .

Getting lost . . .

Where do we get some water?

Why didn't you lose weight before coming to school? You know there's no chance of getting a guy looking the way you do.

My inner critics chimed in, as usual. I opened my eyes. What they said had merit, I couldn't argue that, but I could choose to ignore them. So I did.

Forging ahead, I made my way in what I thought was a pretty straight line westward. Sadly, I did not inherit my papà's sense of direction. His big feet, curly hair (before age turned him bald), sense of humor, affinity for the outdoors, and love of words were what he passed down to me. Oh, how he could turn a phrase.

Italian is a naturally lyrical language, and Papà having lived the first forty years of his life in his hometown of Custonaci, on the west coast of Sicily, just a couple of miles from the Mediterranean Sea, meant he was born into his sing-songy speech not only in Italian but even in his native (and much harsher-sounding) Sicilian. Papà was a poet at heart and set so many of his romantic thoughts of love and life to music whenever he played a tune on his mandolin. Of everyone I had left behind, I knew he would be the one I would miss most. Especially now, when I felt a bit lost, literally.

All around me, all I could see were trees: shady oaks, camouflaged sycamores, hairy white poplars, and familiar maples, my favorites. I couldn't wait to see them explode in yellows, oranges, and reds come fall.

How I could have used Papà right then and there. He was like a human GPS. Growing up, I always knew he could navigate us through anything to anywhere. I never really worried about not getting to our destination; just the opposite, in fact. Papà had taught me that, regardless of our circumstances, the answer was to always move forward with an explorer's heart.

"Chi sa dove va questa strada?" He'd often wonder aloud where some uncharted road would lead, always with a smile and a twinkle in his eye, just before we headed out on the path less traveled. It didn't matter where we ended up. Sometimes it would turn out to be a dead end, and we'd have to go back the way we came. But always, it was the journey—full of feeling, free and joyful—that fascinated us and was so worth our time and effort. Getting lost was part of the fun.

There was only one time in my life I could remember when getting lost for Papà wasn't intended or an accidental bit of entertainment. It was the first time I saw him let his guard down completely, no longer able to hide reality from his children, and saw how he felt when really losing his way mattered.

WE HAD JUST COMMITTED MAMMA to a psychiatric ward. I think we ended up putting her in the University of Chicago hospital that time, but I can't be sure. It was hard to keep track. At the age of fourteen, I had had my fill of hospitals and mental illness and doctors who seemed to know less than I did about the reality of having a mom diagnosed with paranoid schizophrenia. None of the medications seemed to work, although my mamma's refusal to take them had a lot to do with their effect or lack thereof.

Mamma continued to believe in her conspiracy theories—mostly, that the house was bugged and outfitted with cameras that captured her every move on tape. Usually, she saw herself naked, displayed in lewd photographs in national magazines and on the television news stations. And she was convinced her entire family—Papà, my nineteen-year-old sister, Caterina (Cathy), my seventeen-year-old brother Rosario (Ross), yours truly, and even the baby of our family, my twelve-year-old sister Vincenzina (Viny)—were in cahoots with the authorities, and part of a master plan to do her in.

Why did she believe such things? Your guess is as good as mine. Auditory and visual hallucinations are symptoms of paranoid schizophrenia. And in Mamma's case, her mental illness had gone untreated for so long, with one misdiagnosis after the next, that she had become rageful and scary and a threat to herself and others. She kept knives and baseball bats under her mattress and often threatened to kill Papà in his sleep or set the house on fire and take us all out in one fiery blast.

Kill or be killed. That was where we were at in 1979.

When we admitted her to the psych ward against her will, we were told we were not allowed to visit for a couple of weeks. Hospital rules demanded it. And I could not have been more thankful. With Mamma gone, my entire family, for the first time in I don't know how long, slept. The house was silent; the tension, fear, and drama disappeared. And even though we all knew it was just for a few weeks, we rejoiced in it, welcomed it, pretended it would go on forever.

Unfortunately, it wouldn't. On the day we were first allowed to visit Mamma, all five of us robotically shuffled down the hospital's long halls, illuminated by the flood of light coming from a row of hanging pendant fixtures overhead. I guessed that this was similar to walking down death row in prison. We were just as alone, despite being all together.

Surprisingly, while we were there to see her, Mamma wasn't there to see *us*. Somehow, she had disappeared. She was nowhere to be found, either in the hospital or on its grounds. It was as if she had just vanished. Papà was bewildered. We kids were confused. The doctors and nurses on the floor raced around, apologized, and expressed complete disbelief that anybody could slip out of their psych ward, let alone the entire hospital, undetected.

But Mamma wasn't like anybody else. She was extremely intelligent and artistic, a seamstress so talented that when she emigrated from her hometown of Nicosia, Sicily, to the United States at the age of thirty-one in 1958, the famous designer Emilio Pucci commissioned her to sew for him in Chicago. She was also beautiful. When my papà, Antonino, a self-made barber ten years her senior, was on a ship heading toward his own American dream, he befriended Mamma's younger brother, Salvatore, who showed Papà a photo of his still-single sister Maria—Mamma in her twenties—dressed as a mandolin player in celebration of Carnivale. My father loved playing *il mandolino*, and when he saw the young woman in the photo with her hair the color of night, skin as smooth and creamy as a homemade zabaglione, blood-red lipstick—her signature—and curves that filled out that mandolin player's costume, to hear him tell it, he was hit by "the thunderbolt," just like *The Godfather's* Michael Corleone when he first laid eyes on his Apollonia.

But when he learned of Mamma's disappearance from the hospital that day, he became struck by something else: confusion. The man I'd grown up with, who had always found his way regardless of the circumstances, at that moment no longer could.

After spending an hour or so searching for Mamma at the hospital, we gave up and left. After we made our way back to our car and all of us took our places inside, Papà started up the engine and pulled out from the parking spot. We silently inched our way through the neighborhoods of Hyde Park (at that time, the late '70s, not exactly the safest place to be at night). I gazed out the side window, watching the puffs of smoke burp out from the exhaust pipes of other cars on the road. Slowly, I began to realize that we had passed the same houses a couple of times.

I started to pay closer attention. Same street. Same turns. And then Papà stopped the car and pulled over.

Our human GPS had broken down.

"*Ma, bambini, dove siamo?*" Papà, in a very nervous, frightened voice, was asking us where we were.

That shook me to my core. He never got lost. And here, finally, Mamma's madness had succeeded in breaking him. He no longer knew the way.

I SHOOK MY HEAD CLEAR, expelling the memory, and focused on where I was now, my college campus surroundings. I wasn't lost. I was exploring. This had nothing to do with any kind of madness. It was completely normal.

Yeah, but where the heck are we?

No clue.

So many towering trees, sunshine peeking through their branches and playing hide-and-seek with the leaves, creating shadowy figures on the ground: this is what surrounded me. I slowly surveyed the crisscrossing walking paths that stretched out before me, beckoning me to follow. I had already followed them for what felt like miles, and despite having a map in hand, I'd managed to get completely turned around.

"*A volte devi grattarti la testa,*" Papà would say.

At that moment, I, too, found myself doing exactly that— scratching my own head and wondering how to get to my intended destinations: Curtiss Hall and Memorial Union.

I tried to focus. I had promised myself I wouldn't do this— wouldn't think of home or Mamma or my siblings or even Papà while away at school. And here I had been doing just that, which was why, probably, I had gotten distracted and, subsequently, lost.

I thought you said you weren't lost.

I needed to quiet my inner naysayers. How, exactly, I would do that was still an unknown. Keeping that little bit of insanity inside of me at bay was proving more of a challenge than I had anticipated.

This is MY time, far away from all the madness, I chastised the voices.

It hadn't been my time since I turned double digits. By the end of my tenth year, I had already mastered playing the role of *la piccola mamma*. My papà had given me the title of "little mother" and I'd willingly stepped into it, serving as caregiver and *consigliere* for Papà, who spoke broken English at best. In the years that followed, I'd translated employment notices, medical reports, invoices, and school permission slips (writing and signing them for myself and my little sister, too).

Was permission to be just me too much to ask for?

Maybe it was, because, unfortunately, even this short time away was looking as if it would be a financial stretch—and the year had yet to begin. I needed to earn some money while at school, not only for living expenses but also to help make sure I could pay my tuition bill when it was due.

ISU posted what they called "New Student Week Activities" starting the very first Monday morning of the fall session. Designed for those students who couldn't attend the fall orientation that had taken place days earlier, it included campus tours (which, given my current position of having no clue where I was, would have come in handy), and a job fair (which, given my current bank account and the lack of zeros attached to the numbers in it, I couldn't afford to miss). I wanted—had—to be first in line for work-study opportunities, if only I could figure out how to get to the building where those would be offered.

I *would* have been at orientation. I *should* have been at orientation. I *could* have been at orientation. But just days before Papà and I were to drive the five or six hours from Skokie to Ames, a handful of friends had treated me to a farewell lunch at D.B. Kaplan's, a famous deli that sat on the seventh floor of Water Tower Place along Chicago's Magnificent Mile. At the restaurant, many of the sandwiches were named for celebrities, national icons, and recognizable locals. "The Lake Shore Chive," with roast beef, cream cheese, and chives, was my choice. Others ordered sandwiches like "The Studs Turkey," named for radio journalist Studs Terkel, or "The Hammy Davis, Jr.," named for the legendary performer. D.B. Kaplan's was famous and fun and the perfect, festive send-off for my big adventure.

But just a few hours after sharing a laugh and chowing down that day with my friends, I found myself sitting on my bed at home, clutching my abdomen and feeling as if an alien was trying to climb out of it. I tried everything not to disclose how sick I was, afraid of what it might mean in terms of delaying my departure for school. But the pain proved too much, and off we went—my papà and me—to get me poked and prodded by the local hospital's ER staff, who soon confirmed that I had a very severe case of food poisoning.

Delay, delay, delay.

The fear inside me did its best to convince me that this was a sign. Surely, I wasn't meant to leave my family and go to an out-of-state school. Surely, my falling ill was a warning.

I'll admit, I did curse my fate at that moment.

Why me??

Maybe this *was* a sign. After all, who did I think I was? Why should I get to escape the madness? And who else gets ER-level food poisoning on the eve of changing their life forever?

Fortunately, my heart still whispered, "Go!"

And I listened.

I NEVER DID FIND MY way to the job fair that day.

Retreat. Retreat. Retreat.

As much as I wasn't inclined to heed similar advice following the D.B. Kaplan food poisoning incident, I found myself at the moment in agreement with my inside navigation system (or lack thereof). I needed to turn around and head back to the dorms.

Exhausted, sweaty, hungry, and, to be honest, more than a little weirded out that no other human seemed to be on the path I was on, I turned back the way I came and carefully retraced my steps.

Although it had seemed to take forever to get to where I had on the way out, the return trip to my dorm seemed to take no time at all. I was too tired to figure out how that could be, and too grateful to have found my way back to my temporary home to give it another thought—at least until I got showered and changed and drank some water, anyway.

"After all, tomorrow is another day," I said as I approached the concrete residence hall, not realizing I was using my outside voice to say it until it was too late. Most unfortunate to mimic Vivian Leigh's line and dramatic hand gestures from *Gone with the Wind* at the exact moment I crossed paths with a couple of college boys who seemed to appear out of thin air.

Thankfully, they kept talking to one another as if I didn't exist.

I was accustomed to being ignored. I actually preferred being invisible. After all, the alternative—getting noticed in my current, sweaty state, when my ever-present obese physique was already bad enough—could have been so much worse.

I had grown to hate the way I looked: pear-shaped body; curly, frizzy, drab brown hair; plain brown eyes; too-thin lips. I had not enough breasts (and one was a half-size bigger than the other) and way too much butt and thighs. Mamma always said I'd look taller than my five-foot six-inch frame, *if* I slimmed down. Papà always said I'd be a magnet for boys, *if* I just lost twenty or thirty pounds. I was sure they both were right, just as I was sure that wasn't going to happen. I had tried and failed, tried and failed, tried and failed again: Weight Watchers, Jenny Craig, T.O.P.S., even the cabbage diet—which, for a Sicilian girl who loved to eat and who had never before even heard of that smelly, flatulence-inducing vegetable, was a sign of true effort on my part.

Who do you think you're kidding? my inner critics demanded and laughed hysterically. I knew they'd have something to say about my attempts at weight loss. They always did. Sadly, they were more right than wrong.

I had known only one person who could match me for appetite and love of food. God, how I missed her, despite it having only been a few days since I'd left her back in Chicago. Donna was my partner in crime. We'd been best friends since the beginning of high school, and we shared everything. Our struggle with weight topped that list.

Every New Year, we'd talk about how *this* was the year we'd finally do it, even turning our New Year's resolution into somewhat of a cheer: "We'll look fine in 1979," "We'll weigh less than a ton by 1981," and "We'll be free in 1983."

Every January 1, we meant what we chanted. But pretty much before the week was over, our diet plans would get derailed. Sometimes I was the first to fall off the wagon, and other times it was Donna. And when it was her, what kind of friend would I be if I didn't throw myself off the track right along with her?

Such was the case one frigid January when Donna and I had decided to join a local weight loss group called T.O.P.S.—Taking Off Pounds Sensibly. With address in hand, we drove up and down the same suburban Chicago street, searching for the meeting center. Even with the car heater on full blast, it was so cold we could see our breath when we spoke. I was beginning to lose feeling in my fingers.

"Okay, so it's gotta be here somewhere," Donna said as she gripped the steering wheel with one gloved hand, scratching her blond head with the other.

The windows kept fogging up. I tried to help by extending both my hands out to the windshield and using the palms of my mittens to wipe clear a circular scope of visibility. "Let's just park and ask somebody, Donna. I'm freezing."

Donna pulled over in front of the Crain Funeral home. As she did, we saw a trio of portly ladies scurry inside. We both looked at one another.

"This can't be right," we said at the same time, just as we both realized that maybe it was. The T.O.P.S. meeting was held at a funeral parlor. We busted out laughing.

"This has to be some joke," I said.

"Maybe it's incentive," Donna squeaked out, laughing so hard she had to wipe away tears. "Maybe it's like, if you don't lose weight, this is where you'll end up."

We collected ourselves—pulling down our hats on our heads and wrapping our scarves around our necks and mouths so that the only things exposed were our eyes, and then donning our mittens in preparation for exiting the car. Donna turned off the engine, and we both braced ourselves as she opened her door first. A blast of icy air bulldozed its way inside. She struggled to unfold her plus-size, nearly six-foot frame as I hoisted my own roly-poly self up and out of the passenger seat and hurried to exit as best I could. Together, we shuffled quickly along the short walkway, careful not to take a tumble, then pushed open the door and walked inside.

We were greeted by a lonely sign in the lobby. Its little white magnetic letters spelled out "T.O.P.S.—Parlor A." Right underneath it, a second message revealed that a real funeral, for a real dead person, was taking place in Parlor B.

This is seriously messed up.

It was. This was no laughing matter. But Donna and I couldn't shake the giggles, no matter how hard we tried.

We entered Parlor A and managed to weigh in without incident. When we were directed into the actual room where the meeting would be held, however, all bets on best behavior were off. Donna muffled a belly laugh, coughing and nearly choking as a result, as she pointed to the front of the room. I turned to follow the direction of her finger, and my eyes grew wide as they glossed over the dozen or so overweight women sitting on folding chairs, all in a row, and focused on what took center stage at the front of the room: a highly polished, almost metallic-looking, cocoa-colored, closed casket.

What the fuck?

Robotically, we made our way to a couple of seats in the last row and sat down.

"Do you think somebody's in there?" Donna whispered to me, her green eyes glassy from tears, due to both the refrigerator temperature of the room and her attempt to stifle her laughter. I shrugged and held my scarf up to cover my mouth to suppress my own chuckling.

The woman in charge of the meeting, a redhead with an ample bosom and too-tight skirt, kept giving us the stink eye. Then she addressed us directly.

"Ladies, we have a couple of virgins with us tonight," she said.

Donna and I raised our eyebrows and locked eyes. Virgins? The whole room laughed.

"That's what we call first-timers," one woman explained.

I knew what Donna was thinking. Same thing I was thinking. *Weird and true.*

We were encouraged to share our stories, if we wanted to. We both declined. All we really wanted to do was to get out of there. Before we could even come up with a plan of escape, the "angel ceremony" began, during which tiaras were donned by those celebrating big weight loss victories.

Our laughter only grew louder. We tried to conceal it. We knew we were being rude. We just couldn't help ourselves. We counted down the minutes to the end of the hour. But barely twenty minutes into the meeting, neither of us could keep it together any longer, and I slowly raised my hand.

What, exactly, was I going to say? I had no clue.

"Yes, dear, did you want to share something about yourself?" The leader smiled.

I rose to my feet. I could see Donna's look of bewilderment from the corner of my eye. "Ladies, I'm sorry, but we aren't able to stay more than thirty minutes tonight," I said as apologetically as I could. "I need to catch my train to get home." I tapped Donna on the back. "We gotta go now."

It took Donna a second to unfreeze, but when she did, she shot up out of her chair, unable to even make eye contact with anyone or say good-bye, and raced toward the door. I followed. The trail of voices behind us bidding, "Hope to see you next week," escorted us outside.

The minute we exited, we howled, our chortles billowing puffs of vapor in the freezing cold air.

Donna unlocked the car doors. We climbed inside. She started up the engine, and turned to me. "Virgins? Tiaras? A casket?"

"*Twilight Zone* or *Candid Camera*," I said, wiping away tears.

"Catch a train?" Donna laughed even louder.

"I didn't know what else to say, Donna. But I couldn't stand it another second. Did you want to stay?"

"Hell, no." She emphatically shifted into drive and sped off down the road. "Did you ever see that *Mary Tyler Moore Show* episode about Chuckles the Clown?" she asked, once again erupting in laughter.

I nodded, joining in her giggle-fest.

"Mary and Mr. Grant and the whole newsroom go to pay their respects to Chuckles the Clown." Donna could barely get the words out. "He died in a freak accident—he was dressed as a peanut and an elephant tried to eat him. At the funeral, Mary can't stop laughing."

Both of us gasped for air, wiping away tears, trying to compose ourselves. Up ahead loomed the neon-lighted maroon sign we both knew only too well—Baker's Square, the notorious pie house. We had already planned to do dinner after the meeting, but swore it would be on the healthy side.

I couldn't help myself. I had to ask, "Baker's Square? You hungry for pie?"

Donna nodded without hesitation. "I could eat."

"I could eat" became a mantra for us. A private joke we claimed as our own.

Within minutes, we were seated in the restaurant, still laughing and trying not to choke as we chowed down on juicy burgers and greasy fries. Of course, neither of us could have expected what happened next, as in walked the T.O.P.S. leader who marched herself over to our table. We were caught, not only in our lie, but also in our farthest-thing-from-healthy food fest.

Donna breathlessly spoke up, "Her train was early, and we missed it." As plausible as her explanation could have been, her entire demeanor in delivering it betrayed her. No matter how hard she tried, Donna just couldn't lie convincingly.

The T.O.P.S. leader's lips thinned. It was clear she wasn't buying it. With a curt nod, she left us to our own dietetic delinquencies.

Donna and I tried to stifle our uncontrollable laughter with our napkins, but it wasn't possible. Besides, our slices of pie had arrived, and we couldn't very well eat them with our mouths covered up.

That T.O.P.S. experience with Donna pretty much summed up my overall efforts with diet programs. It also spoke volumes about my relationships—with others and with myself.

Codependent! the voices in my head shouted out. And they were right. I knew the word's definition well: "A person with an excessive emotional or psychological reliance on a partner, typically one who requires support on account of an illness or addiction."

My entire existence back home was filled with codependent relationships: my parents' relationship with one another; my papà's with me; mine with Donna. She and I could lift one another up, and we did in many ways. But when it came to diet and healthy eating, more often than not, we dragged one another down, usually without meaning to or even realizing it.

Codependents confuse caretaking and sacrifice with loyalty and love.

I knew it but still fought it. Nonetheless, I did acknowledge that sometimes friends and family had the power to keep you from succeeding at whatever it was you wanted to do. Not that it was their fault. It wasn't Donna's fault that I was overweight. That was all me. She just made it easier for me to stay that way. And I was sure I made it easier for her to do the same.

There's safety in the status quo, even when it's making us miserable and stopping us from becoming everything we could be.

I HAD REACHED MY DORM ROOM—correction, temporary housing/kitchenette. I needed a shower. Badly. I hoped Beth wouldn't be in the room. I could only imagine what I looked like, given I could smell myself with every step. I was super hungry, too. And I imagined that a jock watched what she ate, which meant she'd also be watching what went into my mouth. If I could get into my room, grab my stuff, race down the hall to shower, come back and change, and head out to grab a bite without her witnessing any of it, I would rejoice. I'd already blown my campus map expedition. I needed to succeed at this first-time effort at dorm-life-wash-and-wear-self-care.

With one hand still holding my useless campus map, I grabbed the doorknob with my other. I quickly said a prayer—"Please, God, let the room be empty"—then turned the knob and pushed it open.

I exhaled when I saw that my prayer had been answered. The room, indeed, was empty. Come to think of it, the entire high-rise seemed unusually vacant. I hadn't seen a soul on the elevator ride up to my floor or during my dash down the hallway.

Maybe you're missing out on another orientation thing.

I tried to ignore the thought. I had already missed too much. I may have been an upper-classman, but I felt very lower-class and as if I didn't really belong.

As I grabbed my toiletries, towels, and keys, I focused on the next pressing scenario causing me to freak out: communal shower-ing. The floor had two bathrooms, one on each end of the hallway. The actual toilets had doors for privacy, but the showers were all basically out in the open—only a flimsy curtain that didn't really extend from end to end hung as the divider and one's protector from anyone else who might saunter into the area. I feared being seen in my birthday suit. Even I didn't want to see me in my birthday suit.

I fast-walked out of my room and down the hall, past several real dorm rooms to one bathroom. After stepping inside, I again let out a sigh of relief: The coast was clear.

I practically slid into one of the shower stalls, then hung my towel and change of clothes on the hooks just outside the clingy curtain. Shampoo, conditioner, soap, toothpaste, toothbrush— all of it had to be either juggled in hand or set down on the tile floor. I hadn't thought to bring some sort of hanging shower container. I hadn't thought of a lot of things that would probably have occurred to anyone else. I was still in my street clothes and needed to peel them off and put them somewhere.

Before I could decide what to do, all of the toiletries I had been trying my best to keep in my hand fell and came crashing down around my feet.

"You okay?" A voice that sounded like Beth's echoed in the room.

I froze.

"A couple of us are gonna go down to dinner," she continued, not waiting for a response. "Wanna come with?"

I shut my eyes.

How embarrassing.

She won't rip open the curtain, will she?

Shut up. Focus. She's waiting for an answer.

Okay, so if you say "no" they'll think you're stuck up.

But if you do say "no" then you can take your time putting yourself together and eat without an audience.

"Sure," I heard myself blurt out. I didn't mean to, but it was hard for me to say "no" to anyone or anything.

"Cool," Beth said. "We'll wait for you in the room."

"K," I said, and then, still fully dressed, I turned the handle of the faucet.

You're such an idiot, my inner critics berated me as I tried to stay out of the way of the hot stream of water flowing from the shower head.

I couldn't argue.

Moments later, I managed to strip myself of my sweaty clothes and toss them just outside the curtain. I then tackled washing my hair and soaping up my body. That damn curtain kept getting in my way, groping my ass with every turn. Clearly, the stall dimensions weren't configured for someone my size.

I needed to hurry. Beth and whoever else made up "we" were waiting. With a final rinse, I turned off the water. I waited to see if anyone had entered the bathroom and heard nothing other than the sounds of the shower head dripping and my own heavy breathing. I was surprised by how much effort it was taking just to shower. I assumed I was safe and that no one was lurking outside, waiting to surprise a naked me. But then again, one couldn't be too careful. I opted to dress while still in the shower stall.

WHEN I MADE MY WAY BACK to the kitchenette, I found a note taped to the outside of the door. It read: "Too hungry. Couldn't wait. Meet us at Commons."

I couldn't have been happier.

Juggling an armload of my stuff, I managed to pull off the note, and turn the doorknob to let myself into the room. I was relieved that Beth wasn't waiting for me inside, just as much as I was a bit annoyed that she would leave the door unlocked. She had to know I would have taken my keys. But then again, this was Iowa. Maybe they never locked their doors. And if she had locked it, and I hadn't had my keys, I would have been left out in the hallway with a pile of dirty, wet clothes and an armful of toiletries.

You really need to get your act together.

I know.

And what exactly do you think there is in here of value that somebody would want to steal?

I looked around the room, ready to respond to the snarky chatter that never ceased. Neither Beth nor I had bothered to unpack yet. And what we had still in boxes or bags wasn't anything that couldn't be replaced, at least in my case. Surely Ames, Iowa, had to have a fat girl's clothing store, right? If it came to it.

Shaking my head, mindful of the ticking clock, I threw my stuff onto the floor beside my cot and grabbed the dining card ISU had included in my orientation packet. I had opted for the cheapest meal plan, but it still wasn't all that cheap—hundreds of dollars for the year, and that didn't even provide three squares per day. I was allowed two meals per day, and I doubted it was all-you-could-eat.

Making my way down to the ground floor, I exited my high-rise and followed the short walkway that connected it to the squat building next door, Maple-Willow-Larch Commons. I figured that Larch and Maple were the names of the two Willow clone buildings nearby. Other than that, I had no idea what to expect once inside. Quite frankly, all I cared about was that my dining card held enough credit to handle what the rumbling in my stomach signified it wanted, which was to eat whatever they were offering, and a lot of it. Dinner needed to be served *now*!

After entering through the front door, I scanned the dining room. Groups of guys and girls—some looking so young they might still be in grammar school and some looking old enough to be teachers—stood patiently in lines, trays in hand, waiting for red-and-yellow-uniformed servers to dish out something that, I had to admit, smelled delicious.

Where was Beth? Before I grabbed my food, I needed to know where I would be taking my seat. Was she alone? No, she had said "we" when inviting me to join her for dinner. But did "we" mean one other person or a full entourage?

She was so short that in the sea of seated students, it took me a while to find her. Finally, a hand shot up and caught my eye. It was Beth, still in the same sweats, waving me over. She was seated across from a dark-haired girl whose back was turned to me. I motioned to Beth that I'd get my food and join them. Then I entered the line and accepted what was offered: burgers, hot dogs, French fries, onion rings. I would have taken two of each, but people were staring. I was used to it. Everybody everywhere seemed fascinated by what a fat person ate.

When my tray and I—holding one burger, one small order of French fries, a tall red plastic glass filled with ice and Coke, and a bowl of chocolate pudding—finally got to the table, I could have kicked myself for not grabbing more food. Beth's tray spilled over with doubles of what I had gotten, except instead of Coke she'd opted for milk.

I placed my tray beside Beth's and sat down in the chair next to her.

"Is that all you're eating?" Beth's eyes widened as if in shock.

"Are you really eating all that?" The words came out of my mouth before I could stop them.

The girl sitting across from us laughed out loud. "That's nothing for Beth!"

Beth roared too and then, in the most serious of tones, said, "You'll need to step it up if you want to dine with me again."

My shoulders, which were hiked up to my earlobes, immediately dropped.

"I'm Kathy." The girl put out her hand to shake mine. "Beth and I went to high school together in Brooklyn."

"Brooklyn, New York?" I asked, shaking her hand.

Beth nearly spit out her milk.

Kathy giggled and exaggerated her words. "I wish! Brooklyn, *Iowa*. Have you never heard of it?"

I shook my head and chomped on a couple of French fries.

"It's like an hour and a half from here," Beth explained. "Kathy's family owns Jim and Mary's Café in town. They're famous. My parents have cows. Yup, I'm just some farm girl who's all about eating."

Beth seemed so serious, she made me laugh. She wasn't at all what I had expected a *jock* to be. Maybe I wasn't at all what she'd expected a fat girl to be.

"Where are you from?" Kathy's face lit up when she spoke. "Beth said you're a city girl?" Her big brown eyes sparkled when she smiled.

I swallowed the giant bite I had just taken of my burger. "Chicago. Actually, I was born there, but we moved to a suburb called Skokie when I was little. That's where my family still lives now."

"Skokie?" Kathy wrinkled her nose. "What kind of name is that?"

"Indian," I responded. "I think I was told it means 'smelly onions' or something."

Kathy laughed. "Ewww! You probably aren't missing that, huh?"

I shook my head, smiled, and stayed silent as I savored the last bite of my dinner.

I suppose I could have explained that Skokie didn't actually smell like onions. I could have clarified what I was or wasn't missing. But then I'd have to tell the truth, which was that I wasn't missing home at all. Nope. Despite sharing a kitchenette with a jock, sleeping on a cot, communal showering, and having no clue how to get around campus or whether or not I'd be able to pay my bill at the end of the year, I was at that moment enjoying my freedom from the madness I'd left at home and finally getting a taste of what it was like to be normal.

CHAPTER TWO: **CAMOUFLAGE**

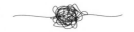

MY PRACTICE WALK FROM THE Willow Residence Hall to the building where the ISU Job Fair would be held served me well. As misguided as I had been just the other day, lost for what seemed like hours, today, when it really mattered, I'd found my way without any delay.

What about the detour to the cereal bar?

While it was true that I had taken the time to eat breakfast in the Commons, I'd done so in great part as a form of research. I had my ISU dining card, and knowing what foods were offered at what times would help me in the long run to budget my calorie intake, as well as my account's piggybank. The fact that I now knew giant dispensers of every possible brand of cereal were on display and available in all-you-can-eat fashion just proved my point.

It also had me feeling so out of control, wanting to grab a bowl of every single kind, just like that terror of a kid Augustus Gloop from *Willy Wonka & the Chocolate Factory*. If you don't remember how the story ended for him, one word: badly. So, while cereal, especially when funds might run low, was definitely on the menu for me, I would have to be mindful of how much of it I consumed. I didn't need any more help resembling an Oompa-Loompa.

As for the Job Fair itself, was I first in line? Heck, no. Scores of students, who I assumed were in similar financial situations to mine, coiled in single file all the way around the building. By the time I approached the counselors at the head of the queue, the open positions that remained weren't exactly what I'd had in mind. Granted, I wasn't sure what that was, but getting paid $3.75 per hour was for sure not it.

Out of all the posted positions, one actually caught my eye: the Animal Ecology Department was recruiting for someone to prepare letters to alumni and write their monthly newsletter. While I wouldn't be working directly with the live animals, there would be opportunities to assist with the birds, frogs, bunnies, and "other duties as assigned."

As I read the job description, I noticed one of the Job Fair representatives smiling at me, widening her eyes, and raising her eyebrows. When I made eye contact with her, she made her way to me.

"Hi, I'm Janet, the Animal Ecology Department's office manager." She nodded at me and moved a few steps closer, so that we were practically nose to nose. She clearly had no concept of or need for personal space.

I took a step back.

Janet's big blue eyes and rust-colored pixie-cut hair made her look more like one of the students than an adult, let alone any kind of authority figure. She looked like such a tomboy. Her stick-figure body was dressed almost from head to toe in faded denim: jeans, jacket, shirt. At the front of her tiny waist, she sported the biggest brass belt buckle showing off a girl riding a bucking bronco. I noticed her steel-toed cowgirl boots and wondered if the belt buckle was a picture of Janet on her own horse. She had to be in her thirties, but she had ridden them well.

I nodded back. "I'm Paolina."

"What's your major?" she asked.

"Journalism and media communications," I responded, even though I wasn't yet solidly committed to it. I had thought about getting a law degree, and for a long time in high school, I'd thought about becoming an obstetrician or even a veterinarian. Unfortunately, every one of those professions required a lot of years of schooling. Who had time for that, let alone the money?

Janet shared more about the job. She needed someone fifteen hours per week. I explained that as much as the work interested me—I loved animals and loved to write—I really needed to make as much money per hour as possible to make it through the school year. To my surprise, Janet immediately upped the hourly wage to $4.00 per hour. It wasn't much, but it was more than the others seemed to be offering. And I liked Janet. She seemed so warm and real.

It was settled. I'd start the following Monday. Just like that, I had a job. I could check that to-do off my list and breathe a little easier knowing that I'd have some money coming in while at school.

NEXT STOP: PAYING MY TUITION for the first semester. No more stalling. I had some grants and student loans lined up, but I still owed a couple thousand dollars. According to the statement the school had sent me, not only did I owe the balance for non-resident tuition but also for an activity fee, a services fee, a building and recreation fee, a health fee, and a technology fee, and let's not forget the room and board fee. I wondered if I could opt out of some of the fees I wouldn't be using, like the fitness center.

You should get a discount since your room isn't really a dorm room.

I would be sure to ask.

Consulting my campus map, I raced across the lawn to Beardshear Hall. The line of students waiting spilled outside onto the building's front steps. I joined this new queue, pretty proud of myself for the day's accomplishments so far. If I hurried, I could make it back to the Commons in time for lunch.

Do you ever think of anything but stuffing your face?

Twenty minutes later, I still found myself in pretty much the same spot. We had barely inched forward.

I tapped the shoulder of the guy directly in front of me. He turned to face me.

"This is the line to pay tuition, right?"

He looked down at me, his eyes peering over the top of his glasses. "Oh, no." He shook his head. "Right building, wrong line. You need to go to the third floor."

"Shit." I exhaled the word. I could forget about lunch, that was for sure.

As I started to walk away from him, he said, "Well at least you didn't spend your whole morning in the wrong line."

Glancing over my shoulder, I smiled and nodded, then raced up the staircase, only to find an even longer line than the one from which I had just come.

By the time I finally reached the clerk who stood behind the counter, two whole hours had passed. To then be told that I was in the wrong line and needed to return to the one I'd been in at the start of my day made me want to kill the boy who had redirected me.

IT WAS LATE AFTERNOON BY the time I had squared away all of my school business. Classes would begin on Wednesday. Even though this was my third year of college, I was being admitted to ISU as a sophomore.

Seriously? So now not only are you losing money, you're losing credit hours, too?

What was the point of arguing—especially when I was doubting my choices right along with the voices?

The classes I was able to get into included an astronomy class on the sky and solar system; a zoology class on basic human anatomy; a journalism class on mass communication; and two English classes, one on propaganda analysis and the other a creative fiction writing course. Five classes plus fifteen hours of work each week, not really knowing a soul, and no one really knowing me—I felt so free. It didn't matter to me that I didn't even fully understand how studying the sky and solar system fit into my degree. I didn't care at that moment if spending all that money and essentially losing a year of education would really be worth it. All I knew was that for the first time in my life, it was just about me, and I could be normal just like everybody else.

THE FIRST THREAT TO MY YEAR of normal came in the form of a letter that arrived just days after I settled into my home away from home. Postmarked August 28, 1985, it was addressed to me, but it seemed so strange, so distant, to see my name and address scribbled on the envelope by my papà's shaky hands.

I sat on my cot, staring down at my own hands and the front of the envelope. I was so glad to be by myself. I really didn't want to be reminded of what I had left behind. Just holding the envelope made my stomach flip. Part of me wanted to leave it unopened so as to stay blissfully ignorant of life back home. They had taken pen to paper to stay in contact with me because they wanted to; I, meanwhile, was trying to figure out how to get out of replying. A sense of obligation left me feeling guilty.

Taking a deep breath, I turned the envelope over, slid my finger underneath the corner of its flap, and slowly pried it open. After pulling out the two carefully folded onion-skin-thin sheets of paper, I smoothed them flat and began to read:

Koku Ⅺ. 8/28/85-

Mia cara figlia Paolina,
Sono trascorsi tre giorni da quando ti ho
lasciato in Iowa; non sono tanti ma a
me sembra come se fosse già un mese.
Vorrei telefonarti ma tu ancora non hai
il telefono, allora quando ricevi questa
lettera telefoni tu (colletta).

"Mia Cara Figlia, Paolina, Sono trascorsi tre giorni da quando ti ho lasciato in Iowa; non sono tanti, ma a me sembra come se fosse già un mese."

My eyes began to well up with tears. Papà had written that while only three days had passed since leaving me at school, for him, it felt as if already a whole month had gone by. My heart sank; I was ashamed at not being able to feel the same on my end, even for him.

"Vorei telefonarti, ma tu ancora non hai il telefono. Allora quando ricevi questa lettera telefoni tu (colletta)."

Ugh. A point-blank directive from Papà saying he wanted to talk, and since I didn't yet have a phone, I needed to call home collect. He continued with a list of questions. He had so many: Did I meet my roommate? Did I find out where to eat? Did classes begin yet? Did I miss my family? Double ugh. The last thing I wanted to do was call home and have to answer the question I knew would be asked: Did I miss them?

The letter continued with individual messages from others in my family. The note from my little sister read:

Hello How are you doing, Don't be scared
To be on your own you can do it
I wish I could do That stay alone I
mean I don't want to go you Know where
good bye Love Vinny.

"*Hello. How are you doing? Don't be scared to be on
your own. You can do it. I wish I could do that, stay alone.
I mean, I don't want to go you know where. Good bye.
Love Vinny.*"

Before I had left for school, it was decided that it wasn't safe
or healthy for my sister to stay home alone all day with Mamma
and her rants. So the "you know where" in her letter was my
Aunt Rose and Uncle Sam's home on the South Side of Chicago.
Mamma's behavior had become too unpredictable and volatile.
As much as Papà had hoped Viny could stay at home and take
care of Mamma, she was just too scared of our mother to be of
much help. It wasn't the best for either of them, so Viny was
being sent to live with Mamma's younger brother and his wife
for a month, if not longer.

I wasn't sure exactly what problem her temporary housing
would solve. Papà had already tried something similar; he'd sent
Viny to Sicily for the summer years prior.

"*E meglio cambiare l'aria.*"

A change of scenery: what Papà thought Viny needed. His
point of view was not shared by Mamma. She objected to Viny
spending time with Papà's older sister and only sibling, Zia
Caterina (or TiTi, as Papà called her). Mamma's objections had
nothing really to do with the money it would take to send her.
And she'd given little thought to the burden being imposed
on our relatives for the extended care and keeping of someone who was pretty much a stranger and not the best at taking

care of herself. No. What was Mamma most concerned about? Appearances.

As a child, Viny was adorable. She shared Mamma's same sleek black hair and wide-set eyes. While Mamma's skin was the color and smoothness of fine porcelain, Viny's was blessed with a rich olive tone that made her look as if she had a year-round tan. As a teenager, however, Viny's love of food didn't sit well on her short stature. The added pounds and her recently permed, frizzy, short hair had turned her into a facsimile for one of those children's toys, Weebles. Only in Viny's case, she had balance issues, which meant that unlike the Weebles, which couldn't fall down, she often did.

Viny was slow, and not just because she was overweight—it was more than that. Her physical capabilities, especially her fine motor skills and coordination, were lacking. She struggled to pick up a penny or correctly hold a pen in her hand. As a result, her penmanship looked like that of a second grader. Ms. Coffee, her actual second grade teacher, had seen signs of Viny's delayed mental and cognitive development, and had suggested to our parents that it would be wise to hold her back a year instead of having her move on to third grade. Ms. Coffee had made the case that without a grasp on the fundamentals of the subjects being taught in second grade, Viny would have nothing to build on and would continue to fall behind in third grade, having no real chance of long-term success.

As logical and compelling as her argument was, it didn't matter. Mamma wouldn't even entertain the thought of Viny repeating the second grade. She saw it not as a way to help with Viny's education and future but as something that would socially stigmatize her daughter and disgrace the entire family. *What would people think?*

Mamma railed at home, punishing Viny for not trying harder and for embarrassing her. Sometimes, the verbal abuse became physical. Mamma's slippers seemed to have some sort of built-in radar; regardless of distance, they could accurately hit any one of us who happened to incur her wrath. Viny promised to do better, but what none of us really understood at the time was that this was the best Viny *could* do. So, unfortunately, Mamma got her way, and Viny continued to pass from one grade to the next, learning nothing and, sadly, becoming more of a target for school bullies to pick on.

The day Viny left home for the airport to fly to Italy, Mamma forced her to wear panty hose that were constricting and so ill-fitting that the crotch hung practically to her mid-thighs. She also made her wear a very tight dress, made of 100 percent polyester, and two-inch heels. Viny wasn't one to ever wear that kind of outfit, but Mamma's choice of attire wasn't for comfort; rather, it was based on her opinion of what a proper young lady should wear. She was trying to make sure that the first impression Viny would make when stepping off the plane wouldn't be that of a rumpled, wrinkled, unrefined mess.

Unfortunately, that's exactly what she ended up being. The fabric didn't breathe and was prone to static build-up, which caused Viny to shock herself no matter what she touched. The added humidity made her hair look like a fuzzy Q-tip and her face, with its sweaty mix of makeup (another thing she never wore), look like it had been painted by Salvador Dali. I could only imagine how uncomfortable she must have been squished into a tiny airplane seat for the thirteen-hour (at least) journey.

When Zia Titi saw Viny emerge from the plane, she called to confirm Viny's landing and chastised Papà for the condition in which she arrived: torn hose (Viny never had learned how to handle panty hose without ripping them) that had cut into her legs; streaked lipstick across her face (she had a habit of wiping her mouth with the back of her hand); and a dress that clung to her, dripping from sweat.

"*Ma, che pensavati?*" our aunt asked. What were you thinking? I wanted to know, too.

It wasn't too long into Viny's visit that Zia Titi called Papà again. This time, it was about much more than just outward appearances. And while she affectionately addressed Papà by his nickname, Nino, her tone of concern could be heard through the receiver as she shouted.

"*Nino, tu figlia non è a posta.*"

Papà's eyes welled up with tears. Zia was right: Viny wasn't "right."

At home, Viny spent much of her time by herself. She didn't have any friends. Anyone who did show any kind of interest in her ultimately took advantage of her. She was frequently the target of others' jokes—or worse. Unfortunately, we all were so preoccupied with Mamma's health and well-being that Viny and her needs went unnoticed. She just seemed to fall between the cracks.

Rosario's contribution to the family letter, on the other hand, managed to crack me up, beginning with his take on silver linings:

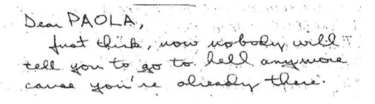

"Dear Paola, just think, now nobody will tell you to go to hell anymore 'cause you're already there ..."

My brother always did seem to find the humor in any situation. He was the only other male in the family, and the only existing Milana heir—although heir to what, exactly, was up for debate, since we had not much of anything to call our own. In our Sicilian household, however, a boy enjoyed so many more freedoms than we girls ever did. So his birthright was to do as he pleased, or so it seemed. Staying out late, bringing girls home, partying in Chicago's downtown clubs ... Rosario definitely took advantage. How could he not? His Italian swagger, *Magnum, P.I.* looks, and quick wit earned him quite a following of females who wanted to date, if not marry, him, and a number of others who wanted to befriend him, hire him, or be him. As a rising draftsman and wannabe architect working for a mentor who specialized in the architectural style of Frank Lloyd Wright, Rosario was enjoying his own idea of normal and all that life could and should be.

Life for my older sister, Caterina, wasn't as happy-go-lucky. I struggled to understand why. From my viewpoint, she had it all: brains and beauty and a degree in marketing from Loyola University. Fiercely independent, she spoke her mind. She worked at a big marketing company close to home that employed lots of people her age, so she never lacked for parties to go to. She had already saved enough money to buy her own car. She loved to dance and had inherited Mamma's shapely legs. Naturally slender, she curved in all the right places and in all the right proportions. Her dark hair and matching eyes turned heads. Her only problem? She didn't know all she was and already had.

I often thought of my sister as a real-life Adrian, the character played by Talia Shire in the Rocky movies. Until Rocky started courting her, Adrian didn't think much of herself. And at the age of twenty-five, my sister hadn't yet found her Rocky, or herself. She sent me letter after letter, sharing her stories of mismatched boys and dating mishaps and repeatedly asking me a question I wondered about as much as she did: where were *our* Rockys? At least she had not yet given up her quest—or her sense of humor.

P.S. In Answer to your Quest.
My Love Life Sucks. Thank you.
How's yours? Probably much
more productive than mine.

One person in the family who had definitely given up any shred of hope was Mamma. Her note to me came separate from the family's joint letter. Papà had written in his that they were headed back to the doctor the very next day to see what else they could do to free her from her demons. In the meantime, Mamma had taken pen to paper to write her own message:

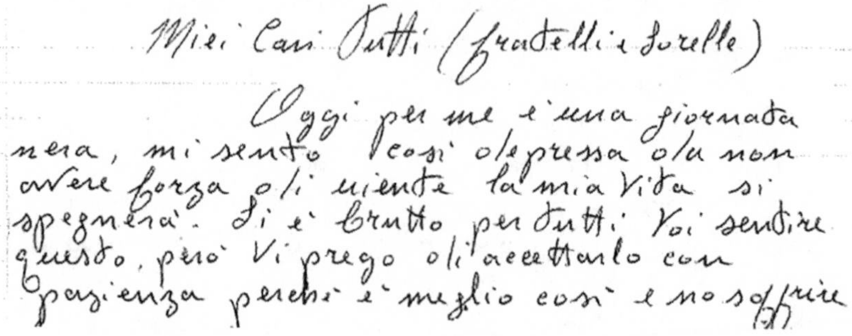

[handwritten letter in Italian]

> Miei Cari Tutti (fratelli e sorelle)
> Oggi per me è una giornata nera, mi sento così depressa o/a non avere forza o/i niente la mia vita si spegnerà. Si è brutto per tutti. Voi sentire questo, però Vi prego o/i accettarlo con pazienza perché è meglio così e no soffrire (?)

"Oggi per me è una giornata nera, mi sento così depressa da non avere forza di niente."

She had written letters saying her good-byes.

"Today for me is a black day, I feel so depressed to not have the strength for anything."

More than just good-byes, the letters seemed to be her attempt to put into words all she was feeling. All she believed she was experiencing. All she had been hiding, perhaps, for her entire life. All that not a single one of us fully understood.

Mamma had battled her demons in silence for decades, until she could no longer keep them quiet, was no longer able to win the wars. Alone and in despair, she'd started coming up with her own solutions to the problem, one of which was suicide.

In Italian, to give birth is *"dare alla luce"*—to give to the light. My mother's choice of words in one of her farewell letters—*"la mia vita si spegnerà"*—illustrated her wanting to extinguish her own light. I marveled at her word choice. Even as schizophrenia stole her spirit and jumbled her thoughts, Mamma's artistry still spoke through the beauty of her words.

"Si, è brutto per tutti voi sentire questo..." She acknowledged how terrible it must be for us all to be hearing this but begged us to accept it with patience because, *"è meglio così e no soffrire"*—it's better this way, to no longer suffer.

Mamma only wanted to escape. I only wanted the same. For her. For me.

I had for years.

Enough! You promised this was your year!

I put the letters back in their envelope and dropped them into one of the boxes I had yet to unpack.

ON MY FIRST DAY AT MY work-study job, Janet took me through orientation. The office was small, but big enough to fit three desks. On top of hers sat a thirty-gallon fish tank, minus the fish. The creatures living in close quarters in the all-glass terrarium must have had their own dreams of escaping. An eight-inch, taupe-colored garter snake and a blue-spotted salamander already shared the habitat. They were about to become *Three's Company*, as Janet held a chubby toad in her hands and was gently lowering him into his new home.

In a deep baritone, she spoke out loud what she was sure the toad was thinking: "I don't know, man. You really think an amphibian like me has a shot with this hot princess?"

She then switched her voice to one that was more high-pitched and responded, "Toad-i-ly!"

I laughed, as did the head of the Animal Ecology Department administration and our big boss, Marie, who had just come out of her office to join us.

"You'll get used to the voices, Paolina," the elegant brunette—who seemed to be paying homage to the 1960s with her bouffant hairstyle—explained. "But maybe not Janet's jokes."

That was funny!

The voices in my own head chuckled at the irony of me getting used to voices. If only Marie and Janet knew.

Strike that. Better that they didn't.

My eyebrows rose as I watched Janet replace the metal lid to fit atop her pets' container. "Hey! You love my jokes, Marie. You know you do."

Marie's eyes peered over her black-and-gold-rhinestone-studded cat-eye glasses. She shook her head and did her best to appear annoyed. But it was pretty clear from how the corners of her mauve-colored lips kept trying to curl into a smile that she was anything but.

Janet concluded her tutorial on how to clean the terrarium, a task that was now mine to do. "You're not afraid of reptiles or amphibians, are you?"

Marie clip-clopped to the desk where I would be sitting and dropped off a manila folder. She once again tried to cast a disapproving glare Janet's way. "Well, I sure hope you would have found that out before you hired the girl!"

"I like snakes," I offered up. "I've never actually held one. I've never even seen a salamander or a toad, other than in pictures, but they don't scare me."

Janet nodded and shot a jesting smirk at Marie.

"And Charlie?" Marie asked in an accusatory tone. "Did you tell Paolina about him?"

I raised my eyebrows again, wondering what kind of creature Charlie was. I envisioned a sleek blue fish with dorky glasses and a little red cap on top of his head.

"Is Charlie a tuna?" I asked.

"Good one," Janet smiled, scrunching up her nose. "Let's go meet him."

Marie turned on her heel, retreating back to her office, while Janet beckoned me to follow her. I fell into step with her as she exited the office, and together we walked out into the empty hallway. We'd only made our way a few doors down when Janet stopped in front of the door to our left and started rummaging in her pockets for keys. She pulled out a jangling ring and fingered a few of the keys before choosing one, ramming it into the lock, turning the doorknob, and pushing the door open.

Even before crossing the threshold, the pungent smell of formaldehyde hit me. I cupped my nose and mouth with my hand.

"You'll get used to it," Janet sang out over her shoulder as she sauntered into the room.

What if we don't want to get used to it?
Exactly.
I walked my way over to where Janet now stood, in front of another oversize door. I looked around at the sterile setting, which was eerily silent, and a chill ran down my spine. I couldn't tell if I was cold due to the actual temperature or if all the chrome and steel made me feel colder than it really was. The room seemed to be the size of two, if not three, standard classrooms. At least a dozen or so metal lab tables, like the ones we'd had in my high school chemistry class, filled the space.

After selecting yet another key from her ring, Janet unlocked what I was starting to realize was some sort of freezer storage unit. I willed myself to stay silent, no matter what was on the other side.

Janet pulled the door toward her with some effort, stepped inside, and quickly emerged again pulling a stainless steel table on wheels behind her. On top of it lay a long black bag with a zipper down the front. It only vaguely resembled a human in form, but I knew that was what was inside.

Janet maneuvered her show-and-tell until it was directly in front of me and then dropped her hands to her sides, the slightest of jingling interrupting the silence. She locked eyes with me and took an exaggerated breath; she seemed to be searching my face for some sign of whether or not I'd need to be carried out on my own gurney. My expression must not have set off any alarms, because without a word, she continued the unveiling.

Her hands reached up to the top of the bag, grabbed the zipper's pull tag, and slid it down to mid-point. She then pulled back both sides of heavy plastic, exposing the head and torso of the cadaver.

"This is Charlie," Janet introduced my new friend, stepping aside for me to get a better look. "Charlie, this is Paolina."
Why aren't we gasping?
That is so gross.
I thought he was fascinating. I couldn't take my eyes off him. Charlie's skin had been peeled away. Nerves and muscles

and ligaments and bones—his insides were exposed. His chest cavity seemed like an empty suitcase either waiting to be packed or unpacked, either preparing to go somewhere or just returning. His soul, clearly, no longer held residence, nor did some of his organs, as best as I could see. They must already have been dissected and studied, I surmised. His lungs and heart, however, were still inside, recognizable and somewhat intact.

"This anatomy lab has classes in here on the days and times you'll be working," Janet said matter-of-factly. "You'll be getting the room set up, including prepping Charlie."

I wasn't sure what "prepping Charlie" meant. I didn't have it in me to ask. I had dissected rats and pigs and even a pregnant rabbit in my St. Scholastica High School advanced biology class. As much as I'd felt sorry for the critters who unwillingly sacrificed their lives for my education, I'd also been curious to learn firsthand about their parts and what made them tick deep inside. But I had never dissected a human being, let alone seen the work in progress.

Surprisingly, Charlie's eyes were the one thing that caught me off guard. I knew he was dead, but his eyes were wide open—or maybe the lids had been removed, I wasn't sure. Whatever it was, his cloudy eyes seemed to still have something to say.

"Are you okay?"

I jumped at Janet's question, lost in my thoughts. I nodded.

Janet zipped Charlie back into his bag. I then helped her push him back into the refrigerated storage.

Shouldn't we have gloves or goggles or a hazmat suit?

I felt the need to wash my hands.

As Janet and I walked back to the office, I couldn't help but think about Mamma dying. Whether it was when she was in a rage because she hadn't taken her meds or when she was in a near catatonic state because she had, it was always her eyes that spooked me. I wondered what hers would look like in the end. Would her beautiful brain, with all of its madness, one day be studied, just like Charlie's body? Would someone find the key to freeing Mamma from her demons long after it would matter for her or her family? Would Mamma's magic reveal itself in her life after death?

I had no clue.

BY THE TIME I RETURNED to my dorm room, the mail had arrived. With it, another letter for me. This time, it was from my sister Caterina. Her elegant handwriting made my temporary housing address look somewhat regal.

"Let me fill you in on what's going on around here," she began.

Please don't.

Are you kidding? Don't you want to know?

The endless battle in my own brain couldn't decide if ignorance was or wasn't bliss.

Let me fill you in on what's going on around here. First, of all mom might be getting out of the Hospital this Friday! Whenever I've gone to see her she seems physically well & at least she's calm. However, you can still tell that she's in a semi-vegetative state (come se dice, e per i nurolle).

From what my sister reported, Mamma had been committed again. Her outbursts couldn't be controlled, which meant that now she would be over-controlled and drugged into submission. Caterina said that when she visited Mamma in the hospital, she appeared much calmer, but also that she was in a semi-vegetative state, describing Mamma as having her *testa tra le nuvole*.

No surprise. Experimenting on people with mental illness by cooking up drug cocktails with no exact recipe to follow seemed to be somewhat of a game show kind of thing for the healthcare community. Never mind if their "a pinch of this and a dash of that" approach didn't seem to be working. It saddened me—not just how clueless those in charge of the care and keeping of crazy were, but how their inability to find solutions meant my perspective on and attitudes about the world had to change. For example, even the words we used no longer held the same meanings. "Cocktail" used to mean a boozy beverage, and while it still did, for me it now conjured up visuals of scientists playing with beakers and Bunsen burners and pharmacists filling prescriptions of measured powders that *might* fix what ailed their patients but, more often than not, only made things worse. Everything, I was learning, had both a light and a dark side to it. With the phrase my sister used in her letter—*testa tra le nuvole*—I could now add this to my list of words that had changed meaning for me, and not for the better. I had always associated that phrase—which translated as "head in the clouds"—as something creative or dreamy or, at its worst, somewhat "absent-minded professor-ish"; now, however, it suddenly took on a whole new meaning—one more absent and definitely dark.

That's what happens when you read these letters.

It was my choice whether or not to read the letters, and while I tried to ignore them, they called to me, begging to be opened. I couldn't help myself.

Caterina continued with her updates: Viny was still living with Aunt Rose and Uncle Sam. Mamma was still threatening to blow up the house with everyone in it. Papà had decided his only choice was to get the family out of there and had sold the house for $112,850. Rosario was helping to find a new place to live, since the deal mandated that we vacate by Thanksgiving or the end of November at the latest.

I paused and rubbed my eyes. Thanksgiving was just a few weeks away.

Resuming my read, Caterina's words hit home.

Really Paula as soon as I save a little money, I'm out of here. A person can not live an unstable life, like this. I feel guilty saying this & also saying that I sometimes hate mom, but I can't help it.

She didn't know how much I had felt the same. It was why I'd needed to escape to school. She also didn't know that I, too, felt confused and guilty, not just for wanting to be free from the family but for having feelings of hatred toward Mamma, even though I knew she couldn't help her mental illness. My guilt also stemmed from the secret I kept, the one that only Mamma and I knew: my actions had been the catalyst for one of her suicide attempts.

I don't know what had sparked my actions that particular day. I was "Sweet Sixteen" (although I had grown more sour than sweet). I'm not even sure I consciously chose to do it; it just sort of happened. Like Caterina expressed to me in her latest letter, I didn't know which way to turn anymore. I just wanted all of the chaos and instability caused by Mamma's mental illness to stop. And I had grown to blame and resent her for whatever happened—whether it was her fault or not.

Thanks to Mamma's all-night rants, screaming to no one and threatening Papà with the baseball bats and knives she kept under her mattress, no one in the house was getting much sleep. Dreamily, my eyes focused inside the cupboard on the blur of antipsychotic and mood-stabilizing drugs Mamma had been prescribed in 1981, two of which—Prolixin and Chlorproma-zine—had become staples of her cocktails. On that day, as I fixed her morning cup of coffee, they also became the base for my poisonous potion as something inside of me compelled me to smash a bunch of them up and add them to her hot drink.

I hoped my brew would prove lethal.

I wanted her gone.

As I swirled the mixture with the spoon and turned to carry it into Mamma's bedroom, we came face-to-face. Without any warning, any sound, there she was. She had been watching me throughout my entire pharmaceutical experiment. I could see it in her haunting eyes.

Whether on purpose or by accident, the cup slipped from my fingers and crashed to the floor. I looked at it and at her, and I ran away. As I raced out the door, behind me, I could not help but hear her softly whimpering my name.

At school that day, I watched the clock tick the day away, dreading the hour when I would have to return home. As much as I stalled, however, at the end of the day, I had no choice.

When I finally did return, expecting to still see the coffee cup and spilled drink on the floor, I found that all evidence of what I had done—or tried to do—had vanished. There was no sign of Mamma, either. And I didn't seek her out.

Around dinnertime, Papà came home. He called out to Mamma, asking her what we should eat. I moved toward my papà and saw the smile on his face and those hopeful eyes cloud over. As he gasped, I turned to see what he was looking at: a disheveled Mamma stumbling out of her bedroom, trying to steady herself at the top of the stairs, just as Viny emerged from the adjacent room.

Mamma's hand traveled from her throat to her chest. Her eyes were panicked. Her slurred words were barely audible, until she clearly articulated the word, "*Ambulanza!*"

In the seconds since he'd first seen her, Papà already had sprung into action, climbing the stairs—just as she started to fall.

My eyes connected with Viny's where she stood, just behind and to the side of Mamma. Viny shut her eyes slowly and tilted her head back a little. I could see her chin quivering as she backed up into her bedroom and closed the door behind her.

Mamma was taken to the hospital.

I wondered that day, as I have wondered almost every day since then, if her attempt at suicide was simply her attempt to carry out what she and I both knew I had started. I wondered if she had somehow salvaged what she had so meticulously cleaned up that day and had taken it after I had left. I wondered if it all was because of me. And I wondered how very evil I must be to be *this* me.

While Caterina and I shared the guilt of hating Mamma, I was suffocating with the shame of actually acting on those feelings and keeping it secret.

Was it reasonable to hope to be normal again someday? Maybe the most I could dream of being was somebody—anybody—other than me.

CHAPTER THREE: **CONFIDENCE**

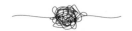

MY STATUS AS A SOPHOMORE and my tardiness in registering for school limited not only the level of coursework open to me but also the availability of those classes; most were already filled to capacity. Given that I couldn't afford to stay in school any longer than was absolutely necessary, I already had taken some of the tests offered through the College Level Examination Program (CLEP). When I learned that I had passed the English tests and would receive college credit for undergraduate work, I felt as if I had just won the lottery.

I never really played the lottery. Papà would occasionally bring home a few LOTTO tickets, and we'd sit around our twenty-five-inch RCA console color TV matching our numbers with the ones called out from the gaming officials. While we never won the jackpot, we cheered whenever we did get even one number. I loved to watch my papà's eyes light up and that gap-toothed grin of his widen. That feeling of excitement of what *could* be—*that* has always stuck with me. Now, having CLEP'd my way into the higher-level, limited-seating creative writing classes, that same feeling of euphoria hit me again.

"Wish I had a million dollars." Jimmy Stewart's character George Bailey, the hero in my all-time favorite movie classic *It's A Wonderful Life*, said that line. Whenever he entered Mr.

Gower's drugstore and soda shop, he would pull on the lever of the old-school cigar lighter that sat on one of the counters. Since the contraption didn't always light on the first try, when it did for George, he'd exclaim, "Hot dog!"

For just a nanosecond, I allowed myself to live in that moment of wishes and magic and the possibilities of what could come true.

And then, of course, I started my usual spiral of worry, wondering when the other shoe would drop. Just as it did for George Bailey, it always did for me.

CLEP, SCHMEP: Passing that test doesn't mean a thing.

Just because you got away with forging tardy slips in high school doesn't mean you can fancy yourself a writer.

How will you possibly hold your own with all of those graduate students?

Who do you think you are?

Fears and self-doubt and the reminder that this, too, shall pass: being normal already was a stretch for me. Ignited from the inside, I felt so much more powerful, something way beyond normal, and, I had to keep reminding myself, way beyond me. When would I ever learn to stop wishing, hoping, dreaming? Doing so only served to wound my heart.

Get out before you get started, before they find out you aren't any good and you fail.

I nearly did drop out, before the first class even began. The only reason I didn't was because dropping classes would have cost me both in academic and financial aid status.

I chose the lesser of two evils.

Sitting in class, however, I wondered if I had made the right choice.

"You all have such fresh faces!" The creative writing professor scanned the room, her playful eyes making contact with mine and, it seemed, every other student's in class. Her bronzed face, framed by more salt than pepper short hair, crinkled as she smiled. Her wrinkles deepened their grooves. In faded blue jeans and a white button-down shirt, its sleeves rolled up to her elbows, she sat cross-legged atop a weathered wooden desk that was positioned squarely at the front of the room. "I'm Lee Hadley," she said. "And I can't wait to learn who you are."

I usually sat at the front of my classes. All through high school and in my first two years of college, I'd race to claim the seat to the very left or very right of the very first row: no distractions—and, if I was honest, I wanted the teacher to see me, to know me, to consider me the best pupil compared to everyone else in the room. But I felt the chances of me being good enough to rank anywhere near the best in this classroom were slim at best. Rather than wanting to be seen and known, I wanted to blend in and stay safe. So the seat I had chosen was at the very end of the very last row: easy access to the exit, should I need to escape.

Professor Hadley shared a bit of her past fifty years living on a farm in Iowa, where she had been born and raised. She made me laugh when she explained a term I had never heard before: "farmer's tan," which referred to the sunburn one got on their neck, lower arms, and bottom portion of their faces—in complete contrast to the pale skin of their chest, upper arms, and top of forehead—due to wearing T-shirts and baseball caps while working out in the summer sun. She told us about her writing career as one half of Hadley-Irwin, having partnered with her colleague, Annabelle Irwin, to write stories that mattered for young adults. Their latest book, entitled *Abby My Love*—a novel about a fifteen-year old, Abby, who had been the victim of her father's sexual abuse since childhood—had just published.

"I guess under this gray hair, I'm still a twelve-year-old girl," Professor Hadley said, beaming.

As Lee spoke, I could feel the fourteen-year-old girl that still lived within me wanting her turn to shout out, "Me too!" I shifted uncomfortably in my chair, as memories of my own sexual predator, Officer Tim Gunner, flooded back.

Gunner and I met at the donut shop where I worked as a teenager. Papà was struggling to make ends meet. Mamma's medical bills were draining. We needed money. I managed to forge my birth certificate convincingly enough to get the job when I was just thirteen years old.

Gunner was thirty-nine. He towered at a slender but muscular six feet. He had strawberry-blond hair, the bluest of eyes, the most Cheshire Cat–like smile, and the swagger of Clint Eastwood, whom I loved.

As I thought back on him, the jumbled feelings of my youth churned in my stomach and that familiar turbulence of arousal, excitement, dread, unease, and shame filled me. It was no use trying to focus on what Lee was saying. Her voice had faded into the background and was now replaced by Gunner's calling out my name . . .

"POWWWWleeena . . ."

From the first time I served him coffee and watched him lick his lips after devouring his favorite strawberry-frosted raised donut, I felt drawn to him—both thrilled and afraid. Something inside tried to warn me of the danger, as much as it also egged me on.

"Do me a favor, would ya?" he asked so innocently the first time. He needed help ridding his uniform of cat hair.

I nodded without understanding how, exactly, he wanted me to help.

He rose and came over to where I stood, joining me *behind* the counter. He had always maintained his distance until that day. Then, suddenly, he didn't.

I watched, unable to think, let alone speak, as he began pulling lengths of Scotch tape from the dispenser, the one we used to seal donut boxes by the dozen. He hummed some unrecognizable tune as he hung each foot-long strip of tape on the top edge of the glass showcase counter, letting them dangle like the streamers that hung off the handlebars of the bicycle I rode when I was little.

He reached out and pulled both of my hands toward him. He lifted my arms and bent them at the elbows, and then positioned my hands in front of his chest, as if he would be placing handcuffs around my wrists. With one of his hands holding one of mine, he took those long strips of tape—sticky side up—and began wrapping them over and over my hands, from the tips of my fingers to the base of my palms.

"I need your help in getting rid of 'the evidence,'" he said, smiling. He arched his back a little and swung his torso from left to right, showing off his body.

That's what he called the mountain of gray cat hair that always was visible on his navy police uniform: "the evidence."

I felt paralyzed, and puzzled as to what I should do or say.

Gunner placed my taped-up hands, palm-side down, onto his chest. His hands guiding mine, he began to use me to stroke him.

"Thank you for helping me with my pussy problem," he said, dragging my hands over and over again down his chest, then his arms, then his thighs. When they became full of cat hair, he'd stop, replace the tape on my hands, then continue, even turning his back to me and asking me to get the backs of his legs and his buttocks.

I did as he wanted. My hands were at his mercy. So was my mind. He taught me how to stroke nearly every inch of his entire body, under the guise of ridding him of cat hair.

It didn't last long—not that time, nor all the times that followed. Nor the night he went too far.

The pain of that memory jolted through me as if it was all happening again, bringing me back to the present.

Breathe. Focus.

It took me a minute to realize where I was. Looking around the classroom, I hoped no one noticed my mental departure.

Lee still sat atop her desk. I wondered if I could tell her what happened to me. I felt she would understand. It was similar to the topic of her book and its character, Abby.

Father Tierney should have understood.

It hadn't gone well at all when I tried to tell my parish priest about Gunner. Father Tierney had refused to hear me out, unless I promised to show up for church every Sunday. I should have just lied and said I would. Being truthful resulted in him refusing to absolve me of my sins. I needed to remember the lesson of that day. Sometimes, speaking up just wasn't worth it.

AS I MEANDERED MY WAY through ISU's campus, the trees' waves of red, orange, purple, and yellow leaves seemed to nod their approval to me. I had finally learned how to get from point A to point B without a map in hand. Now when I got lost, it was on purpose.

Perched on one of the top steps of Beardshear Hall, I leaned back, basking in the autumn sun, letting it warm my face. Lunchtime for me now included taking a seat with a view of the 110-foot-tall tower that stood in the center of ISU's campus. Intrigued by what was called the Campanile (the Italian word for "bell tower"), I had learned that it was built as a memorial to the school's first Dean of Women, Margaret MacDonald Stanton. Her husband, Edgar Stanton, had inscribed quotes on each of the first ten bells. Now it had fifty giant solid brass bells, and listening to them play out their daily noon-hour greeting was like being at an outdoor concert. And even more dear to me was the fact that the Campanile's first few bing-bongs sounded just like the bell-ringing opening credits of *It's A Wonderful Life*.

The Campanile was said to be a love story. The school paper wrote that to be a true Iowa Stater, you had to be kissed underneath the Campanile at the stroke of midnight.

Fat chance of that ever happening to you while you're here.

The voices in my head still enjoyed their commentaries, never letting me forget that they were present. That said, I knew they were feeling defeated. They had quieted considerably, realizing their diminishing power to ruin my moments of joy.

I wondered what the ten quotes on those first bells were that Mr. Stanton had written to his late wife. They probably couldn't have been a lot of words. *How would they fit a long quote on the face of a bell? How big did they say those bells were? If I were a guy, I'd write my girl poetry.*

Papà wrote beautiful poems. Those were love letters, the kind I hoped I'd one day get from somebody who loved me as much as he loved Mamma and who would stick with me "in sickness and in health."

The stack of letters from home sitting in my backpack, waiting to be read, came to mind. I had a bit of time until my writing class with Lee Hadley started. I hated to interrupt my moments of peace with what usually turned out to be more crazy. But if not now, then when?

I repositioned myself so I was sitting up straight against the cool concrete step behind me, grabbed my bag and rested it between my feet, and reached in. I rummaged through my books and folders and notepads until my fingers felt the envelopes, still sealed. I pulled out three at random, placed them on my lap, and began to tear open each one's flap.

They had come all at once: a backlog of back-home news that I would have preferred to remain in the holding pen they had been contained by until this moment. Anywhere else was better than them finding their way to me.

The silver lining of living in temp housing—and moving all of the time—was the delay that it caused in delivering my mail. I was relieved that I did not receive these updates from home on time but dreaded the stack that would catch up to me at some point in my own version of musical chairs. I longed to finally get settled and stay put in a room where I could not only unpack once and for all, but also fully decorate and maybe even consider calling my room "home"—even if it would only be for the seven or eight months remaining in the school year.

ISU had been trying to find permanent placements, ones that didn't include a sink and cleaning supplies, for those who had gotten stuck in temp housing. Beth and I had recently moved out of our kitchenette and into real dorm rooms, but we'd been separated, both of us assigned to new roommates and three-person dorm rooms. It wouldn't be until we were moved a third time that we would end up in our own two-person dorm, together again—this time by choice.

Who would have guessed you and the jock would hit it off?

I was as surprised as anyone. Beth wasn't like anyone I had ever known, at least not in terms of a jock. The stereotypes I believed had convinced me that jocks were judgmental jerks, below average when it came to brains, ate very little and worked out a lot, and usually swung for the same team in terms of sexual preference. While it was true that several of the softball players were lesbians, that wasn't true for Beth. And none of the other assumptions I had made described her either. She was smart and kind, and while she did work out frequently to maintain her enviable muscles, especially for such a tiny girl, she also ate like a grizzly bear storing up reserves in preparation for hibernation. Compared to her, I was the one who ate like a bird. And we were more alike than we were different.

Unfolding Mamma's latest letter to me, I wondered if I had wrongly judged her as well.

"*Carissima Paola*," she began; her salutation of "Dearest" might as well have read, "My most judgmental daughter." Ugh.

I wasn't sure I could read on. What was worse: Having letters that confirmed the crazy back home? Or what I had now before me—letters that cast doubt on my perceptions?

I scanned the next few words, all of which seemed so "normal," with Mamma saying she hoped I was well and settling in.

Sounds normal to us.

I couldn't disagree, but as normal as they may have been to anyone else, they just didn't fit with what the other letters communicated and with what I knew to be true about Mamma. Her next few lines further took me by complete surprise.

"Non ti dico che piango perché sono dura a piangere, però ti dico sinceramente che ti penso sempre."

Mamma wasn't demonstratively affectionate. Even before the schizophrenia consumed her and the drugs suspended her spirit, she'd never been the kind of woman who cried at the drop of a hat or who showered you with kisses when you came home from school. Life had taught Mamma to steel herself against showing others how you truly felt. She had learned somewhere along her own journey that big girls weren't allowed to cry. So to read her words telling me, *"I'm not going to tell you that I'm crying, because crying doesn't come easily to me,"* and to have her not only acknowledge that fact but also confess that what she *could* say to me is that *"in all sincerity"* she *"thinks about me always"* moved me.

Mamma's silence, her keeping secret the voices she heard, the phantoms she swore were real, the isolation she endured, and the depression she must have felt all contributed to her not getting the help she needed at the start of her disorder. She knew she couldn't be the mom she wanted to be, and the mom we wanted her to be.

Memories of a fourteen-year-old me helping my papà commit Mamma to a hospital psych ward made me shiver. Even worse? Holding in my hands her letter of love to me and recalling how relieved I was to be rid of her ate at my soul. I kept my mamma at arm's length, afraid of the demons she battled and the parts of her she could not control. I had closed my heart off to her, and yet here she was, sharing her feelings of love for me in this letter. Had I made a mistake? Maybe, just as I had misjudged jocks prior to meeting Beth, I had been misjudging Mamma all this time? *It's not like you didn't have good reason.* I agreed. I did. In some of her worst moments, Mamma had convinced herself that I had been sleeping with Papà and Rosario. It was then that I'd become the focus of her fury. Mamma had always assumed I was promiscuous. I'd never understood why. And her believing that about me had made what happened with Gunner even worse. Her misjudging me had contributed to my lingering doubts regarding the role I'd played in what had happened that night.

Returning to her letter, reading her final few lines, put me a bit more at ease. I was comforted by what I had become accustomed to; in fact, Mamma reminding me to *"fare sempre la brava ragazza"* actually made me chuckle. *That* was much more like the mamma I knew, the one I often feared, the one I had escaped. Her telling me to "always be a good girl" lessened the guilt I had felt just moments earlier and had me shaking my head, somewhat amused, since I knew that with the way I looked, I had no choice here at school *but* to be the "good girl" she thought I wasn't.

I did a double take at Mamma's closing. She ended her letter with a word I had never before seen or heard her use—*bacioni*, which translated in English to "big kisses"! I had to read it more than a few times just to make sure that was what it said. Yup. Big kisses. Oh, how I would have loved to have been with *this* Mamma at the moment she wrote down those words.

The Campanile's bells continued to ring. I had lost track of how many tunes had played and what each one was.

This always happens when you read the letters.

The words typed on the front of the next letter's legal-size envelope looked as if they'd been hammered out using something similar to the 1965 Olivetti Studio 44 manual typewriter my uncle Joe, Mamma's brother, had given me when I was a teenager. That "portable," breadbox-sized reincarnation of a steel anvil often inked-in certain letters, appearing exactly the same as the letters in my Iowa address stamped on the front of the envelope. The "o" was always the worst, looking as if its inside was shaded in gray on purpose. I could see that the "n" and "y" in the spelling of "University" had been typed over without first being erased. I knew how much force was required to press down on those keys, and yet I loved the thing. Obviously, so, too, did Mr. Austin, my pen pal, who'd written this letter.

His salutation of "Dear Nasty Neighbor" had me howling.

October 8, 1965

Dear Nasty Neighbor;

I think it was real nice of you to drop me a line to see if I was still living; I do appreciate it, possibly more than you think.

You ask in your letter how I was and how I like my new home. The answer to both questions is BAH!!!. In the first place, you probably knew anyway, I'm now living alone, just me and MacIntyre, and I don't like it a bit. Mrs Austin just decided she would rather live up in Waukesha with her daughter. You ask me why? I really don't know, Paula. There was nothing like a scandal or anythin like that and I just don't know way. It's strange, with me being so cute and everything.

I know also that things aren't so good with you family. I was talking with the O'Brines last week and they said how bad your Mother is feeling lately. All along I was tainking how much she had improved, and now I hear just the opposite. It's disheartaing too see a family breaking up, first my own and now yours. So I guess neither of us will have any trouble putting on a sad face for Halloween. I was especially sorry that Vinny ad to quit her job to take care of her Mother. I had heard how nicely she was doing and how she liked her job so much. At least I hope you get a good price for your home but any price will never compensate for you Mother's health.

Paule, I do wish you and your family the best, and I do want you to kiss them all for me. Tell them all I love them and will add them to my prayers from now one.

Be good and try hard in school,

Mr A.

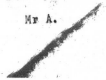

Mr. A, as I called him, lived in the big white corner house directly across the street from our home in Skokie. I guessed him to be at least eighty years old. He had a wife and children—a total of five, I think, but they all were grown and living their own lives. Mr. A was the grandfather I never had. He and his long-time companion, an Airedale terrier almost as old as he was named MacIntyre, would putter around the outside of his home, always waving hello to me and more often than not, walking across the street to sit with me on our front stoop and talk a bit. He always called me "Nasty"; his definition of the word was one of empowerment, as in "don't take any shit." No matter what was making me cry inside, Mr. A could always make me laugh.

His letter confirmed that he now was living alone, no longer in the home across the street. As sad as I felt for him, he still could lighten my mood with his words. When explaining in his letter Mrs. Austin's reasons for choosing to live with her daughter rather than with him, he quipped, "There was nothing like a scandal or anything like that, and I just don't know why. It's strange, with me being so cute and everything."

I thought he must have been quite a character in his youth. He still was. And whether or not Mrs. Austin wanted to live out her days with her husband, I was grateful to have had him as my adopted grandpa.

I was never really sure just how much the neighbors knew about Mamma and all we were going through. We were taught that what happened in the family, stayed in the family. Our unspoken Sicilian family code of keeping secrets was mandatory. It was clear, however, from Mr. A's letter that others *did* know something was wrong, and that they were just as confused about what, exactly, it was.

That was the trickery of mental illness, I had come to realize. One moment would seem perfectly normal, with all systems stable, and in the very next second, crazy would come for a quick visit—or for an extended stay. Keeping people in chaos and constantly off-balance was its specialty.

"It's disheartening to see a family breaking up, first my own and now yours. So, I guess neither of us will have any trouble putting on a sad face for Halloween."

As I folded up Mr. A's letter and carefully slid it back into its envelope, I made a mental note to visit him during my very next trip back home.

The Campanile's ringing had gone silent. I needed to pack up and head to class. I figured I could walk and read at the same time, especially one of Caterina's letters. Her penmanship was clearly legible, even when on the go.

As I gathered my things, I tore open the envelope, pulled out its contents, and gave it all a quick scan.

> Everyone is okay, except guess who. Mom seems to have her ups & downs. However, about a week ago things were definitely on their way down. She refuses to cooperate by taking her pills and she is constantly talking about senseless things.

Nothing much had changed, except I wasn't there to help. Caterina's letter contained a laundry list of to-dos; clearly, she had taken over duties as our family's *consigliere* in my absence. All that I had been to Papà in terms of writing letters, keeping bill collectors at bay, dealing with doctors, and anything else related to communicating in English had now fallen to her, while Rosario was helping to find a house and secure a mortgage.

Also enclosed were credit card bills. My ever-growing mound of debt: Sears, MasterCard, Marshall Field's . . . each statement she had included was one more reminder of all the money I owed that I did not have or have a clue how to get.

I inhaled deeply, shutting my eyes.

Tomorrow is another day.

Scarlett O'Hara's line of hope had become a constant mantra of mine. I decided it best to not read the rest of the letters yet. I exhaled and opened my eyes, then shoved the letters back into my bag, lifted it and myself off the steps, and walked as quickly as I could to join Professor Hadley and the rest of my creative writing class.

It didn't take me long to make it to the classroom. Already, the other students were seated, pens and paper at the ready to record wisdom Professor Hadley had to offer. I slid into my seat at the back of the room.

Professor Hadley hopped up onto the top of her desk, crossed her legs, and looked out at us. She smiled, nodded, and made eye contact with each of us. When she looked at me, I wondered what she could see in me.

"So I gave you all an assignment," she began. "I asked you to write me a short story from the perspective of a gender that's the opposite of yours. I gotta say, you are a creative bunch! But I knew that the minute you all stepped foot in my classroom."

I smiled at her, listening, or trying to, as I absent-mindedly doodled in my notebook. Money was on my mind. How would I be able to pay those bills?

"While all of your stories were great, there was one story that really hit the nail on the head. I'm gonna read it to you now . . ."

Professor Hadley cleared her throat. I kept up with my abstract artwork and worrying about my finances, or lack thereof.

"*It Ain't Worth It!*" she began.

"This was my first time. I couldn't believe I was doing it. But as the old saying goes, desperate situations require desperate actions—and this was a desperate situation."

It took me a second to quiet my internal chatter and focus on the words she was reading aloud.

"I hadn't had a date in months—to be exact, two months, three days, and, by a quick look at my Timex, ten hours, thirty-two minutes, and some seconds of which I had no

idea since $19.95 for a watch doesn't get you a sweeping second hand."

Oh. My. God. Those words were from *my* story. Professor Hadley was reading my story to the whole class.

"I had become the joke of the dorm. I could just hear my buddies laughing at me, 'Hey Skams, maybe you better change your sexual preference—you might have better luck getting a date.' Ha-Ha-Ha. I'd just laugh it off, pretending that it didn't hurt, but it did. Somehow, some way, I had to get myself a girl."

I couldn't stop the spread of my smile. I tried to look to my left and to my right without moving my head. Did anybody realize she had chosen me? That her favorite story was mine?
How in the world would they know that?
She didn't name the author, dummy.
At that moment, every cell of my being pulsed with glee. On the outside, I tried to keep my cool, but my smile refused to cooperate, betraying me to everyone who bothered to look at my face. I could only imagine what Professor Hadley must have seen as she continued to read the words I had written: my Joker-worthy, goofy, giddy grin that I was sure now extended well beyond my ears and clear to the back of my head.

At the end of her reading of my short story, Professor Hadley hopped off her desk, whirled my paper in the air, and presented it to me, saying, "Well done, Paolina!"
The entire class applauded and congratulated me.
I couldn't tell you what happened afterwards in class on that day. My mind kept reliving the experience and was fixated on the "A" Professor Hadley had written on the last page of my story, along with her notes: *Your character never slipped with a voice all his own that was funny, rather dear, and totally appealing to the reader; You should try selling this story to a teen magazine that uses fiction.*

Selling it? Seriously?

She actually thinks it's good enough for somebody to want to buy it?

Disbelief was now laced with something I had never even thought to entertain as a possibility. I could be a writer. Scratch that. I *was* a writer. In that moment, I wasn't just normal or good enough but *better than*—well above average. And for the first time in my life, I realized I just might be able to earn a living as a writer.

CHAPTER FOUR: **CALM**

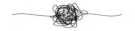

THANKSGIVING BREAK CAME TOO early for me. While everyone else on campus seemed to be hurrying to wrap up their class assignments and pack up their long-weekend bags, I took my own sweet time. Nearly half the year was already over, and I had only just begun to really breathe on my own. Divorcing myself from the madness at home and feeling free for the first time in my life was at risk of getting derailed . . . *if* I was to head home for the Thanksgiving week holiday.

Fortunately, I had an out. It was the one time I'd ever considered my lack of finances to be a blessing. I didn't have the funds to make it home for both Thanksgiving and the upcoming, much longer Christmas break. Plus, there wasn't much of a home to go home to since the Skokie house no longer belonged to us, and Thanksgiving weekend was targeted as the moving date for my family to schlep all of our stuff to the new house Rosario had found and Papà had bought.

When my family learned that I wouldn't be coming home for Thanksgiving, the letters arrived telling me I would be missed. Viny's note from home made me laugh the loudest. While her penmanship was clearly getting worse, her message was clear. Food was a big deal for us.

*I'm sorry it is not tradition To have Pasta fina fina
on Thanks giving what you have is "Turkey," Stuffing
mashed potatoes gravy garlic bread Rolls apple Pie cheese cake
Vegetables fruit and other deserts — ice cream for christmas
Pasta meat and others newyears Day & Eve Love V don't get sentimental*

She listed out anticipated menu items for the big day. Her letter reminded me that in addition to a stuffed bird, mashed potatoes, and all of the traditional American favorites, our Thanksgivings included pasta and other dishes of an Italian flavor.

Not that I ever complained.

Nor did Viny, who closed her note with encouragement for me to "not get sentimental" about what I was missing.

She was probably right. I would miss the food.

UPON LEARNING OF MY HOMELESS holiday situation, Beth graciously offered to house and feed me for the week of Thanksgiving while we were on break from ISU.

"What do y'all typically have for Thanksgiving?" Kathy asked over breakfast in the Commons on the last morning before the campus closed down for the holiday break.

"What does *everybody* have on Thanksgiving?" Beth snorted in between bites of her food.

"Well I don't know," Kathy replied, giggling.

"Actually, we have lasagna," I said, quickly followed by, "in addition to the normal stuff like turkey and stuffing and mashed potatoes."

"See?" Kathy beamed.

"I want to go to your house for dinner!" Beth added.

No, you don't.

"Oh, wait! You're coming to mine." She feigned forgetfulness.

"My grandma always makes chicken and noodles," Beth said exaggerating the licking of her lips. "So close to pasta!"

I smiled as best I could, grateful to have somewhere to go, while at the same time terrified at the idea of spending not just

Thanksgiving Day but the entire week with Beth and her family at their farm. I had never been allowed to attend sleepovers as a kid. I had no idea what to expect, how to act, what to wear . . . the list went on and on.

"We'll have to take you out on the town in Brooklyn, *Iowa*!" Kathy laughed.

"You should take her to your folks' place," Beth added.

"Your parent's house?" I asked.

"No, Jim and Mary's Café," Beth said. "I told you, it's one of Brooklyn's hot spots."

"Oh, Beth!" Kathy giggled. "My parents have a little diner. We'll go one of the days you're out by us."

ALTHOUGH BROOKLYN, IOWA, WAS ONLY a ninety-minute drive east of campus, when we actually rolled into town, it seemed much farther. It was as if we had been transported back to Mayberry, USA, circa 1950. Having come from Skokie, with a population well over 60,000, Brooklyn's total count of less than 1,500 people felt way too tight-knit. I immediately thought of how it would be impossible to keep mental illness hidden in such a tiny town. Everybody had to know everybody else's business. How could you not?

The spit of a downtown alternated between industrial, warehouse-looking buildings and low-level brick-and-mortar shops. Private residences, most of which looked a bit abandoned and had gray siding that could have used a good scrub, were peppered throughout. The typical post office, hair salon, bar, grocery market, hardware store, and bank all seemed cut from the same brown-brick cloth and sort of blended one into the other. Giant silver metal contraptions resembling silos that had lost their pencil-like figures rose up plump from the ground in places they seemed not really to belong. The old brick church with the eighty-foot bell tower, ironically named St. Patrick's, made me think of the cathedral of the same name located more than 1,000 miles east; however, there was no mistaking this one in Iowa for the one in New York.

I would be given a proper tour of the town later. It was onward to Beth's family homestead first.

While Papà and I had driven past lots of farms on Route 30 on our way to ISU, I had never really given much thought to the fact that families actually lived on these farms 365 days out of the year. Beth's family lived on a real working farm. When we turned off the country road and onto the little dirt driveway that led to their house, I couldn't believe the size of the property. It was huge—and with the unusually cold and wintery weather, the snow on the ground made it look like a giant wasteland that had suffered through some nuclear blast. I wondered what it must look like at the height of summer. Towering green cornstalks probably provided a most fantastic maze within which to get lost. Giant, rolled-up bales of hay most likely dotted the fields like lazy sunbathers basking in the sunshine. This was Beth's backyard. I chuckled thinking of my papà spending countless hours after work tending his garden of tomatoes and zucchini and peppers and basil and onions and garlic, and all else that flourished in our backyard, all 300 square feet of it. What he would do with this amount of land, I could only imagine!

I followed Beth into the house, lugging my overnight bag with me. While the temperatures outside were frigid, the moment I crossed the threshold into their living room, I immediately warmed up from head to toe. I peeled off my outerwear while Beth called out to whoever might be around. The inside looked just as I imagined: country through and through. The La-Z-Boy chair and the overstuffed couches were draped with Afghan throws. The hardwood dining room table seemed as if it had been in the family for generations. A fresh polish made it shine—awaiting, no doubt, to be set for the Thanksgiving feast.

In a way, the complete silence made me think of my own home. That's not to say it was the same kind of quiet; rather, it was just the opposite. Quiet back home felt ominous, as if the next tick of the clock would bring doom. Here, however, the stillness brought a sense of calm. Even meeting Beth's mom and dad further added to the feeling of tranquility. She was tall and slender, with short, dark blond, curly hair and wire-framed glasses, while he sported dark hair, chubby cheeks, and a bit of a belly, just like my own papà. From the moment we exchanged hellos, I felt welcome. Their ease and deliberate mannerisms, even in how they took their time speaking and listening to what I had to say, it felt so comfortable, as if hosting orphaned strangers was a daily occurrence for them.

On the other hand, for me, actually embracing the status of "orphaned stranger" or even as "sleepover guest" didn't feel quite so natural.

I had become an expert of sorts at pretending, so I faked it. As uncomfortable as it was, I lounged around in my flannel jammies along with Beth and the rest of her family. I tried to just "hang" and "chill," as much as it was killing me not to "do" and "worry"; there was always something to do and to worry about back at home.

How do people live this way?

I had no answer. But I did have a question to counter. *How come we can't live this way?*

A COUPLE OF DAYS LATER, Beth and I met up with Kathy at her parents' café. Located at the intersection of Country Road V-18 and Highway 6, it was the place for truckers and other motorists to stop for a home-cooked treat. Actually, it was the *only* place around that I could see from that busy road. Kathy drove up in a pickup. She was such a girlie girl, so pretty and joyful. Behind the wheel of that truck, she added fierce and independent to the list of why I secretly wanted to be her.

Kathy offered up anything on the menu, on the house.

How cool would it be to have your own family restaurant?

And be able to do what she just did?

What if we ordered one of everything on the menu?

I shook my head at my mind's lack of manners, although I did want to taste it all. Maybe it was the farm air or just being out with these two farm girls, but whatever it was, I felt more

famished than usual, and not in the "fill me up 'til I'm numb"
kind of way.

Kathy suggested we start with pancakes.

We love pancakes!

Moments later, she placed the oversized plate in front of
me. The three pancakes that sat on top were literally the size
of Frisbees. I could see, too, that they weren't the dark brown,
dry-looking flapjacks one might expect from a roadside diner.
Nope. They were light in color and super moist-looking, and
glistening with a big old dollop of creamy butter. Real maple
syrup added the finish to what looked almost too good to eat.
But eat them I did.

Kathy and Beth's eyebrows hiked up their foreheads as they
both laughed out loud.

"Oh, my God, Paolina!" Kathy exclaimed. "You inhaled
them. You're worse than Beth!"

I hadn't realized how quickly I had gobbled up the pancakes
until Kathy made her comment, and I looked over at Beth's plate,
one she still hadn't finished lapping up!

"Impressive. I'm usually the one who's ready for seconds
before anybody else is," Beth joked.

I shrugged. I didn't know how else to respond, other than
to say, "Those were the best pancakes I've ever had in my entire
life! What's your family's recipe?"

Kathy laughed even louder and put her right hand over her
mouth, as if she was about to spill some secret. She then blurted
out, tears forming in the corners of her eyes, "They're from a
box mix!"

"No way!" I shook my head.

Kathy rose from her chair. "I'll show you." She raced back
to the kitchen and returned with a yellow, brown, and white
five-pound box of "General Mills Complete Pancake Mix" in
her hands. "See?"

I took the pancake mix from her and read the box. "It's completely generic," I finally declared, completely dumbfounded.

Kathy nodded with a grin.

Beth let out a loud, "Ha!" and then nearly shouted, "If you think that's awesome, you're going to love where we're taking you to tonight."

"Where's that?" I asked, now joining in the laughter.

"Only the second-hottest place in town," Beth offered up. "Second, of course, to Jim and Mary's Café."

THE "SECOND-HOTTEST PLACE in town" happened to be The Legion Hall.

"What is this place?" I asked as we drove up to park in front of a very plain-looking, warehouse-like storefront with one big window looking in and lots of loud music booming out. A line had started to form, full of people of all ages, colors, genders, shapes, and sizes patiently waiting to get in. The sun had already set, and it seemed as if the entire town had decided to pack itself into what was more commonly known to me as the local VFW hall.

We exited the pickup and were making our way to the back of the queue that had formed in front of the hall when I noticed Beth's mom, dressed in blue jeans, black flats, and a dark wool winter coat that fell just above her knees, at the start of the line. She threw back her head, laughing with others in line, and I could see her feet already seemed to be dancing, keeping pace with the beat of the music, perhaps, if only to help keep warm.

Her mom?

I tried to imagine Mamma going out to the local bar, but I couldn't. It just wasn't something she would even think of doing.

How do you know?

Know what?

That Mamma wouldn't love to go out for a drink or to hear some music?

I didn't know. And suddenly I wondered if maybe that was some of what Mamma needed.

Back before I had left for ISU, while working in the Bridal Registry at Marshall Field's & Co., my coworker Mrs. Minta had made a comment to me that I'd never forgotten. "B," as we all called her, was such an elegant lady, with not a single blond hair on her head out of place, and always dressed as if she were attending a ladies' luncheon. Though she was well into her forties, her figure was model-perfect. Pencil skirts and pastel cashmere sweaters with a colorful silk scarf pop of color draped about her neck and shoulders were as much her signature as Mamma's blood red lipstick. When I shared just a bit about my mamma's illness with B, she knowingly raised an eyebrow, cocked her head, and said, "I know what's wrong with your mamma. She's got a case of 'dead-ass-itis'!"

Once inside, I watched as Beth's mom juggled a drink in one hand while making her way to the center of the hall's crowded great room. She moved to the music, bopping her head back and forth, and stamping her feet, dancing like a teenager to the pounding sounds of the British rock band Dire Straits's "Money for Nothing."

"Your mom is really good," I shouted to Beth, barely able to hear myself over the near-deafening ZZ-Top-sounding guitar riffs playing.

"It's her favorite song," Beth shouted back, nodding proudly.

What's Mamma's favorite song?

I thought about it. And I had no idea.

The realization that I didn't have any clue about who Mamma was as a person stayed with me long after leaving the Legion. I felt in that moment as if I knew more about Beth's mom than my own. Even as Kathy and Beth and I drove around town for the rest of the night, with Kathy purposefully shutting off her headlights and doing donuts in her truck on dirt roads and in parking lots—and scaring the shit out of me—I couldn't shake how the only things I associated with Mamma were those that had to do with her mental illness. I knew more about what she couldn't do because of her health than what she used to do when she was healthy, and maybe what she still wanted to do but no one among us was taking the time to help her figure out a way to still do them.

You're talking in riddles.

Am I?

And you're not supposed to be thinking of home, remember?
Right.

ON THANKSGIVING DAY, I JOINED Beth and her family for their feast. I don't remember a single moment of it. At some point during the visit, Beth's mom made an incredible German chocolate cake, but I don't think it was part of that day's meal. I'm not sure what was served, not even what Beth's grandma's chicken and noodles tasted like. No clue about who or how many people were there, either.

The table was set, I'm sure. Grace was said, no doubt. People gave thanks and reminisced, I assume. But the thing that I *do* remember is the feeling of peace and tranquility—to the point of my memory erasing all else. That, and of this being how normal families gathered together. Maybe the sharp contrast to the commotion of my own family's feasts is the reason I've blocked it out. I couldn't say.

The other thing I remember is Beth's parents letting me use their phone to call long distance back home. It took a few tries, but I finally got through. My family said they were so busy moving, they really didn't have time to talk. And I was grateful not to have to.

UPON RETURNING TO ISU and heading back to my school routine, I tried to focus on my priorities: final projects, final exams, final bills. That, of course, became a challenge as soon as I got my mail.

Mr. Austin's postcard was waiting for me when I got back to my dorm.

"Always stay nasty." I laughed as I read Mr. A's recommendation to me aloud. I knew he was joking, but by the same token, he was right. I had to steel myself against caring for anybody other than me. I had gotten better at being nasty, but not good

Dear Nasty;
          I was delighted to hear that
you're doing so well at school; an A average
is something to be very proud about and, believe
me, I'm very proud for you. Keep us the good
work, but remember, always stay nasty.
          I wonder where you're family is now living.
You had mentioned that they had to vacate your
house by November 21. I did get a card from Kathy
but she didn't indicate what you were all going
to do. I suppose a lot depends on how your Mother
is feeling. I'm afraid to ask and I do pray that
she might be showing some improvement.

          Say hello to everyone and I still love you
                                             A

enough. A few days spent with a normal family where the kids
weren't expected to take care of the parents and where the parents
actually had fun on their own just further underscored how *not*
normal my family really was. If I wasn't careful, I could easily
slip back into my role as *la piccola mamma,* caring for everybody
else other than me. And with Christmas break on the horizon, I
knew I could get stuck in the swirl of cray-cray that had become
my norm. It was up to me to break free and live my own life as
a normal, "nothing to see here" kind of girl.

As I sat at the desk in the room I shared with Beth, I looked
up at the bulletin board hanging on the wall in front of me. Photos
of Papà and Mamma, my siblings, and my late-uncle Joe stared
back at me. I had pinned them up to remind me of home and the
people I couldn't help but love. Like it or not, this was my family.

I also had stuck in the very center of my photo collage a
greeting card an anonymous somebody had sent me a few years
earlier. The front of the card depicted a colorful cartoon draw-
ing of the word IT as if the two letters combined had been given
life, mimicking that of a menacing human being. IT's features
included bulging eyeballs, an intimidating expression, a threatening stance, and Mickey Mouse–like hands and feet that seemed

hell-bent on doing some damage. IT was shown standing on a welcome mat, huffing and puffing and pounding on somebody's front door, threatening to knock it off its hinges. Flipping open the card, however, the inside message was clear about what the visual intended to communicate: "Don't Let *It* Get to You!"

But it is getting to you.

Don't you wonder who sent you that card?

Other people know the truth about you. You need to do a better job of keeping crazy secret.

I didn't have time to even respond. The second letter that had come in the mail was one from Mamma. I held it in my hands, giving it now my full attention. Postmarked just days before I had headed to Beth's for Thanksgiving, the single sheet of ruled notebook paper was filled on both sides with Mamma's handwriting.

I could feel her rage. With every staccato stroke of her pen, her fury grew. She punctuated her schizophrenic thoughts about the grand conspiracy, her husband's collusion, and her dignity becoming collateral damage. Mamma wrote to me about being taken to a new doctor named Bernstein on November 20, just days before Thanksgiving. She shared how the doctor had asked if Mamma had been taking her pills, to which she replied that she had been. She wrote that Papà had betrayed her by pulling from his jacket pocket her prescription bottles for the doctor to examine. This Dr. Bernstein then counted the pills, one by one, proving that Mamma hadn't taken a single dose since filling the prescription weeks earlier.

Mamma was mortified at being called out for lying. Even worse, her not taking those pills resulted in the doctor, with Papà's approval, giving Mamma an injection of her medications to ensure compliance.

In Mamma's eyes, she wrote, all that had happened that day was further evidence of Papà setting her up to do her harm. While she hated to inform me, she continued, she felt I needed to know that the truth was that Papà was in on the scheme for the medical community to experiment on her—which, in her scrambled state, included them taking photographs of her naked and posed in lewd positions. She surmised that that was why she had been forced to lower her pants in front of the new doctor for him to take an unusually long time administering the shot with the medication—all so that the camera could take her pictures.

Nothing to see here, the voices mocked. Mamma must have thought I would be coming home for Thanksgiving, and assumed that her letter would reach me before leaving ISU for Thanksgiving break. It hadn't. But she wouldn't have known that. And I could only guess that in her confused mind, me not even acknowledging the letter's existence had only further served to confirm her suspicions and fears that her entire family didn't care about her and was bent on exploiting her and doing her harm.

Don't let It *get to you.*

I laughed out loud—probably, if anyone was listening, as close to crazy sounding as one could get. Luckily, I was alone.

Always stay nasty.

After folding up Mamma's letter, I hid it with all the other letters that had come. They shared space in a shoebox alongside receipts to fast food drive-ins and ice cream shops and bars and other places I had no business frequenting—not if I was actually trying to lose weight and save money. The box also kept my mounting credit card bills that were yet to be paid, and anything else I needed to keep secret or that I really didn't want to think about. Not now. Not yet. Not until I absolutely had to.

I stared down at my mound of misery, crumpled messily inside my box. For now, my priorities were all me: wrap up class projects, focus on finals, and finish registering for next semester. I inhaled until my lungs could take in no more and held it.

Right! Who cares about all your mounting bills?

You do know that you can't get your grades if you don't finish paying this semester's tuition, right?

I exhaled sharply, picked up the cardboard lid, and slammed it shut on top of my secret shoebox. Period. End of sentence. I refused to think of it any more.

CHAPTER FIVE: **CAGED**

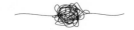

AS MUCH AS CHARLIE NO LONGER creeped me out, he did have me wondering about who he was. What secrets had Charlie kept throughout his life? We all kept stuff hidden. What was his stuff?

Every time I wheeled him in and out of his holding pen, I wondered more and more: Did he have a family? Or did he die all alone and end up here because there was no place else for him to go? Was he sick? Or did he drop dead without warning? As much as Charlie was physically exposed, with all of his nerves and muscles and organs showing, what the students working on him would never know were the things he had kept to himself, deep inside, while still alive.

Had Charlie gotten a chance to spill his secrets before he died? Did God know before or after he ended up here?

Maybe getting dissected like some lab rat was his punishment for the secrets he kept?

Did Charlie's daughter or son, if he had a kid, get to find out what his favorite song was before it was too late to ask?

His favorite song? I just shook my head: So many questions, and too late for them to get answered.

I positioned Charlie in his usual spot at the front of the room. Class would soon begin, and all eyes would be on him. His eyes stared straight up to Heaven. I looked up, wondering if he was looking down on me at that very moment.

"Paolina."

Janet's voice startled me. Like a spooked cat, I jumped, and Janet laughed.

"Don't do that!" I yelped, catching my breath.

"I'm sorry, hon." Janet walked over to Charlie and me. "You want to try your hand at something less dead?"

I furrowed my brow and shrugged. "Sure."

Seconds later, Janet had led me to one of the other large classrooms.

"This is a red-tailed hawk," Janet explained, gesturing to the creature inside the transport crate. "Ever seen one?"

I shook my head, immediately enamored with the great bird inside her cage.

"Well, you're going to get up close and personal now with this one." Janet presented a large leather glove. She nodded, gesturing toward my left arm, her fingers waving in a "gimme here" kind of way. I turned myself over to her, as she fitted me with the thick heavy armor that covered my entire hand and extended almost up to my elbow. "This is so our friend here doesn't dig her talons into you."

"Wait. I get to hold her?" I could barely contain my excitement. This was so much better than working with a corpse.

"I wouldn't call it 'holding.'" Janet laughed. "Think of yourself more like a tree branch she'll use as her perch."

Janet slipped another leather glove onto her own left arm and used it to retrieve the bird from its enclosure. As the hawk flapped her wings and used her beak to gently peck at Janet's protected arm, a few tiny feathers broke free from her wings and gracefully floated to the ground.

She was beautiful. From head to toe, she stood nearly two feet or so. Her neck and chest and belly were a creamy, coffee-colored swirl sprinkled with cinnamon. On top of her back, a mark that looked like a white "V" blended into a mocha tint with darker brown and black flecks that blended into the tips of her wings and tail feathers. And when Janet finally lured her fully out of that cage, the hawk stretched out, spreading her majestic wings, and I swear they spanned a good four feet from end to end.

I gasped, and my mouth stayed wide open in awe.

"Alright now," Janet cooed to her unhappy captive. "Settle down. You know the drill." Little leather straps, almost like tiny leashes, hung from the bird's legs.

Swallowing and forcing my mouth to form the words, I asked eagerly, "What do you want me to do?"

Janet carried the hawk away from its cage. "You'll be at one end of the room, and the Professor will be at the other with our friend here. He'll then let go of her so that she can fly across the room and land on you."

"No way!" Long after the words popped out of my mouth, I still couldn't seem to bring my two lips back together to close my piehole.

"Way," Janet replied, chuckling.

Janet explained that the bird had been found near the side of a busy highway, unable to fly. Her right wing had been fractured, and she had lots of other issues. Usually, the veterinary students would mend fallen prey good as new and get them back out into the wild, but this particular bird would never be able to fly in the wild again. Her injuries had been too severe, and her chances of survival out on her own were slim to none now. So she lived here at the vet school in an outdoor sanctuary. And throughout the school year, she served as a show-and-tell live learning tool and unofficial pet, just like Janet's snake, toad, and salamander.

"Ready?" Janet shouted out from across the room.

I stood with my suited up, leather cast arm jutted out to my side, strong and steady, as she had instructed. "Ready!" I shouted back, bracing myself.

Janet released the hawk. I inhaled and held my breath—
and, standing as still as I could despite the electricity that jolted
throughout my being, marveled at the hawk's movement. Her
wings stretched out and those eyes laser-beam focused on mine;
I was mesmerized. That sound, too—more than a flutter, something I had never heard before, a powerful, repetitive WHOOSH
that seemed to fan her whisper onto my face, almost as if she had
blown me a kiss just before landing on my arm. I expected her
to be heavier than she was, but she couldn't have weighed more
than a couple of pounds.

"Keep your face away from hers," Janet warned as she walked
toward me.

I leaned back, but I couldn't turn away, kept staring into
those piercing amber eyes. She looked so angry, as if this wasn't
what she had signed up for. I couldn't blame her. I knew what
it felt like to be caged, all the while hoping for the chance to
break free.

"She likes you," Janet squealed. "You know, you're good
with animals. You ever thought about becoming a vet?"

As Janet carefully transferred the hawk back onto her own
leather-wrapped arm, I answered, "Actually, I did back in high
school. I loved my advanced biology classes, but honors chemistry did me in. I barely scraped by, got a D."

"*Honors* chemistry?" Janet asked, emphasizing the course's
elevated title.

"I know." I shrugged. "But my school was pretty small, and
they needed one more kid for the class to be a go. I was the
dumbest of the smart kids, so lucky me."

She laughed. "Too bad." She crossed the length of the room
again with our hawk along for the ride and kept talking. "I must
have fallen off my horse hundreds of times. Never gave up. Now
I show horses."

I again took my stance to give the hawk a place to land.

"Ready?" Janet asked.

I nodded. And locked eyes with the hawk.

JANET'S HORSE STORY AND THAT HAWK drove me straight into the Registrar's Office the very next day. I had already signed up for my spring semester classes; Professor Hadley had encouraged me to take her next writing class, so I'd enrolled in that. I'd also managed to get into an advertising principles and a media law class. Two more communication classes were on my schedule, but the thought of spending my one and only year, the last semester of it, caged up like that hawk just didn't seem right. So when I learned that Iowa State University offered a horseback riding class for credit, it was a no-brainer; I rearranged my schedule—dropping one class and keeping the non-verbal communication one—and signing up for horseback riding.

Really? Doesn't that put you behind in credits?

Doesn't it require an additional fee?

I ignored what was correct on both counts. Reading aloud from the course catalog—"No horseback riding experience required"—I almost hugged myself. The fact that the class was under the physical education umbrella thrilled me even more. Me? *Choosing* to take P.E.? Look how far I had come!

Delusional.

Irresponsible.

I signed up, despite the truth of their words. Then reminded myself of one more word I was determined would describe me: free.

THE NEXT FEW WEEKS FLEW BY. Final projects were turned in and final exams were taken. I don't recall any of those final fall semester moments. My thoughts were consumed with the fear of returning home.

When I had talked to Papà on the phone, asking him if anyone might drive out to get me, he said it wasn't possible, and I should find my own ride home. Rosario said that there were lots of ISU students from Chicago who put up flyers on the bulletin boards in the Commons, offering transportation, especially over Christmas break. Surely, I'd find somebody I could pay to share a ride.

I'm sure I could have, but I chose not to even look. The fear of risking any kind of further connection between my normal life at college and the chaos of home was too great. It was much safer to take a Greyhound bus, even though the trip would be a very uncomfortable, long, overnight ride.

By the time we arrived at the terminal in Chicago, the sun was struggling to make an appearance. It would not win its battle, giving up way too soon, conceding the day to ominous gloomy clouds. The moment the bus driver opened the door, I grabbed my bag and was the first one off. I paused momentarily. I had no idea where I was. Everything from the sky to the buildings to the pavement looked dirty. It was as if all the color in the world had been taken out of existence, leaving behind a dull, slushy gray.

I looked up at the street signs: Harrison and Jefferson, an intersection somewhere in the South Loop. I still hadn't a clue. According to Rosario, I needed to walk to Union Station, about a half-mile away, to catch a train destined for a place called Barrington, the closest stop to Algonquin where we now lived. When I got there, I was instructed to find a pay phone and call home for someone in my family to come pick me up.

It was one thing to have to take a Greyhound bus home for Christmas break. Was it too much to ask to have somebody pick me up at the Chicago station? Had we still been living in Skokie, the drive would have been maybe twenty to thirty minutes versus what it was now from Union Station to Algonquin: a good hour, if not longer. That said, it really did surprise me that I had to figure out how to get home—a home I had not even seen—on my own. Did my family no longer miss me? What must be going on, I thought, for even my papà not to show up? Didn't they realize that this part of Chicago wasn't exactly safe for a young girl? How bad must things at home be?

I pulled my coat tighter around me, hugging myself in the process. As I made my way down more streets—Jackson, Van Buren, Quincy, Adams—getting lost no matter which way I turned, I tried to focus on all the names of former presidents that seemed to be the theme of the downtown street signs. With every step I took, my breathing sped up, increasing the foggy puffs of smoke that formed in the air before me. Between the cold and the slight panic, I quickly gave up on my self-imposed history lesson. I never much had enjoyed reliving the past, despite the fact that I often did.

The hairs on the back of my neck started to stand at attention. I wasn't quite sure why, since the entire area was deserted; not another living soul was in sight. It truly looked like the set of a sci-fi flick: a modern-day ghost town caused by some apocalyptic quarantine mandate. Empty buildings of mostly gray concrete lined the sidewalks. Something about them seemed so harsh and menacing. I tried to control my shivering and not dwell on the one word that kept coming to mind: abandoned.

Where are you going?

Someone could jump out from anywhere and grab you.

What's that?

I started to panic, and I pushed myself to get off the narrow sidewalk path and walk smack dab in the middle of the street, wondering where the hell that train station might be.

When I finally found Union Station, I realized I had passed it more than once. It reminded me of when my papà had lost his way, driving around the same blocks that night Mamma escaped from the hospital. I hoped this wasn't an omen of what I would find at home.

From the outside, the building looked like any other that day: cold, hard, the very opposite of welcoming. Once I was inside the train station, however, my eyes widened at the very unexpected marble floors and walls. Corinthian columns stood guard around the perimeter of a Great Hall that soared high over me, opening up to a skylight above. Old world, gold-toned iron scrolls hung overhead: "To Trains" they directed, and I followed.

The sight I encountered upon entering the platforms where the trains were waiting startled me. So many lanes, and so many clones of trains—I had no idea which one was the right one to board.

"Excuse me," I had no choice but to ask the first person that walked nearby. He barely broke his stride, obviously in a hurry to get to wherever he was going, but managed to point his finger at a sign listing all of the destinations, each one's time of departure, and the lane to head to for boarding. Barrington wasn't listed. Of all of the options, the only one that made sense to me was the "Northwest" train. I knew that wherever we had moved to, it was in that general direction. Luckily, that particular train was leaving in just a few minutes. Unluckily, that meant I had no time to double-check. I made my way to the track indicated, boarded the train, and hoped for the best.

That word came to mind again: abandoned.

Where is everyone?

I wondered too.

I made my way to the corner end-car seat. This definitely wasn't like the trains I had been on before. My commute between Skokie and the University of Illinois at Chicago for the two years prior to transferring to Iowa State University had included a combination of bus and train rides totaling about ninety minutes one-way, on a good day. I didn't so much mind the time; it allowed me to peacefully transition from whatever was happening at home to my school work. I did mind the masses, many of them unwashed and unkept, and it always seemed as if the smelly ones would choose to sit by me.

Now in this new kind of train that was taking me to Barrington, not only did I find myself cradled comfortably in a very clean and cushioned seat, I also quickly found the need to remove my outer layers, almost baking from the car's heated interior. The doors remained open, too, long enough for passengers to exit without scrambling and with frequent announcements on the loudspeaker of when they would be closing. It all seemed so luxurious and courteous.

Just a few moments later, the double doors slid shut and we jerked into motion.

I looked around. The entire car was empty, except for me.

Where is everybody?

I kept asking myself that; I felt so exposed. In that moment, I would have preferred the sardine packing of the city's subway system to this "last human standing" sense of abandonment.

Just then, the train's conductor entered through the door that connected the car I was seated in with the next one. In his blue uniform and pill-box hat, he made his way down the empty aisle, squeezing and clicking the hole-puncher in his hand.

"Ticket?" he asked when reaching me.

Shit. You never bought a ticket.

What an idiot.

"I'm sorry," I stammered. "Does this train go to the Barrington station?"

He sighed, blowing out a salami-smelling breath of air. He pulled slips of paper out of his pocket, punched holes in them, and then handed one to me. Then, without uttering a single word, he continued on his way, sliding open the door of our car, disappearing into the next, and letting it shut behind him.

I don't know why he didn't charge me for that ticket. He couldn't possibly have known that I didn't have the money to pay for one. No matter the reason, I felt a sense of being cared for—by who or what, I didn't know. And I didn't need to know. For the first time since leaving Iowa, I relaxed and enjoyed the surprisingly smooth and silent ride. I gazed out the windows, watching the concrete cityscape dissolve into green grasses and open pastures and . . . horses! I envisioned myself back at ISU sitting high on top of some majestic beast. We'd be galloping in slow motion, the wind blowing my hair . . .

"Miss? Miss!" A brusque voice jolted me awake. I could still hear him but couldn't quite make out his words. I shook my head like a wet dog drying itself. My eyes focused outside. Suddenly, I realized we had stopped moving.

"Barrington?" The train conductor stood over me. "This is your stop."

I jumped up out of my seat, so embarrassed. I must have fallen asleep during the ride. Awkwardly, I collected myself and my luggage, struggling to stuff myself back into my outerwear.

"Yes, thank you," I stammered as I made my way out of the train. I also silently thanked God for this guy who'd not only paid for my ticket but had also remembered my destination and come to check on me.

Who does that?

Did you thank him for the ticket?

I had just stepped off the train and onto the platform. I turned back to address the conductor, but the doors already had closed and the train was set in motion.

A honk-honk from behind me drew my attention. I turned back around and there in the parking lot in a cream-colored 1978 two-door Mercury Marquis sat Rosario. With one arm out the open driver's side window, he waved me over. Clutching my bags closer to my body, I jogged over to the passenger side, pulled open the back door, and tossed them onto the backseat. I shut that door, and then opened the front one and folded myself onto its seat.

"You made it!" Rosario said. He rolled up his window and put the car in drive.

I turned to look at him, and then immediately burst into tears.

Why are we crying?

I had no answer. I hung my head as low as I could get it toward my lap.

Rosario chuckled. As he turned the wheel with his left hand, easing the car toward the parking lot exit, he grabbed my left shoulder with his right and gave it a shake. "Hey! What you choose to call hell, we call home."

His laugh was contagious, and soon I couldn't help but follow. I shifted from bawling like a baby to giggling like one, asking, "What the hell is that supposed to mean?"

"Rambo," he replied, as if the answer was obvious. "Didn't you see it yet?"

I shook my head.

"Oh, I forgot." He laughed. "I-O-W-A isn't exactly a premier showing city, is it?"

I shrugged.

"Anyway, that's the best line," he said. "And it fits, doesn't it?"

I shrugged again, wiping away my tears with the back of my sleeve. "How did you know to show up? I was supposed to call you."

"Clearly, your time in the Iowa cornfields has warped your mind," he joked. "Have you forgotten? I know everything."

"Right!" I scoffed. Turning my face toward the window, I silently redirected my attention to the little shops and the people that made up this town called Barrington. Christmas lights swirled and shoppers blurred as we sped on by.

"It's not that bad," Rosario said.

I half nodded, keeping my gaze outside. "The house? Or Mom?"

"Both. You'll see."

We continued without much talking. He turned up the volume on the cassette tape he had popped into his car's stereo. Tapping his fingers on the steering wheel to the song—it was called "In Between Days" and was by some band called The Cure, he informed me—he shared that it had become his favorite tune.

"Never heard of them."

"Are you kidding me?" He exaggerated his response to the level of shock and horror. A moment later, he returned to pure Zen. "Oh, right. I almost forgot where you've been for the last several months."

As if on cue, The Who's "Teenage Wasteland" began to play.

I turned to look at him, raising my eyebrows and trying not to laugh. He shook his head, muttered "tsk, tsk, tsk," and then reached up to his visor, pulled down his Tom Cruise *Risky Business*–worthy Ray Bans, and slipped them on. Lowering his head and peering over the rims at me, he shook his head and said, "Such a waste."

I rolled my eyes and turned my attention once again to the world outside while on the way to my new home. The start of a long white picket fence suddenly came into view. It matched the color of the fallen snow threatening to bury it. An army of weeping willows stood guard at its gates. They must have been cousins of the ones on ISU's campus—similar, but not quite the same. These seemed so much taller, rising maybe fifty feet up into the overcast skies. They also seemed much lonelier, as if segregated from the other species, not at all like the family of different trees that lived together on ISU's grounds.

As I contemplated the treetops, a flash of something not so white entered my peripheral field of view. I straightened up in my seat and twisted my body to the right for a better look.

"Horses!" I cried out as I pressed my left cheek and nose against the chilly glass to watch the two brown beauties trotting through the snow as if they were trying to catch up to us at the end of the fence. We were moving too fast, however, and they never made it to the edge.

Rosario momentarily turned down the music's volume and turned his head to see what I was seeing outside my window. "Oh, ya. There's cows, too." He faced forward again and returned the music to its earlier levels of loud.

Maybe your brother's right: This isn't so bad.

Hey, you can learn to ride horses and come back here when school's over.

I didn't want to think of the day when my one year away ended. Not yet. So for the rest of the way to our new home, I envisioned myself back at school with *those* willow trees and *those* horses and the life that, at least for a little while, was mine and mine alone.

Twenty minutes later, Rosario slowed down the car to a crawl. The street sign said "Homestead" as we turned into the driveway on the corner lot. I sat up a little straighter in my seat. My eyes took it all in. While it wasn't as big as Beth's farm, not by a long shot, the property was big enough to fit at least two of our Skokie homes inside its perimeter.

"Wow!" I nearly whispered. "Big yard."

"Dad's happy." Rosario smiled as he rolled the car to a stop right in front of the two-car garage's white door.

"The house sort of looks like a barn," I said as I pulled on the car's door handle to exit.

"It does not!" Rosario barked. "The rooms are smaller, but overall, it's bigger than the old place." He tried to sound optimistic. "More places to hide. And mom's not talking about torching us all while we sleep any longer."

I rolled my eyes. "Progress!" I mocked his enthusiasm while stepping out and reaching into the backseat to pull out my stuff.

Rosario didn't turn off the engine or make any moves as if he would be joining me. "Aren't you coming in?"

He shook his head. "Can't. Places to go, people to see."

My brother had kept himself out of the Skokie house as much as possible. Now, at the age of twenty-three, with school and a job in the city and a steady girlfriend, why would I think things would be any different? When asked, he always said he was working, and whether he was or wasn't, nobody seemed to be bothered about his whereabouts. Clearly, it was one of the privileges of being a male in a Sicilian household.

As he pulled back out of the driveway, I shouted after him, "Hey, *Rocky IV* just came out." I had hoped he might want to see it with me. But I never got the chance to ask. He rolled down his window just enough to wave a few fingers of his left hand at me, and then, without any other response, he sped off down the street. I stared after him until I could no longer see the back of his car.

I loved Rocky. So did my brother.

"Paulie, you ain't nothin' but a dirty, stinkin' bum," I mumbled to myself; it was one of our favorite lines from the original movie. My brother would always say it to me in his finest Rocky Balboa voice. Rocky was one of his heroes, just as he was mine, but for different reasons. Ever since Rosario had seen the movie back when he was fourteen—its story about the underdog who triumphs against all odds and especially its charging theme song—something had changed in him. He'd become focused, driven, and confident. Maybe he'd been at just the right age for it. Just after the first movie came out, his fascination with Rocky had led him to purchasing and using boxing gloves, a punching bag, a speed bag, and I'm not sure what else. And he'd started running at night:

seven-minute miles. I knew they were seven minutes because he often took me along. I'd ride my bicycle behind him, huffing and puffing, just trying to keep up.

Mamma hated when my brother and I went out anywhere together. In her schizophrenic mind, she always envisioned the two of us entangled in some forbidden sex act. She thought the worst of me in that way when it came to my relationship with both Rosario and Papà. I still didn't understand what I'd ever done to make her think such terrible thoughts about me.

As much as I didn't miss Mamma's accusations, I did miss those days with my brother. Now, my siblings and I all seemed to be doing our own thing, with each of us surviving independently as best we could. For Rosario, that meant having his girlfriend and job *and* keeping his distance from home as much as he could. Unfortunately for me, for the next few weeks, keeping my distance would be near impossible.

It's only three weeks. You've survived longer and much worse.
I nodded. Resolved.

As I made my way up the six short concrete steps that led to my new home's front door, I scanned the neighborhood. Every house around us looked like the same cookie cutter raised ranch. Even the color schemes copied one another. Our siding was the color of brown poop.

The front door swung wide open, nearly clipping my shoulder, as my papà did his best impression of Tigger from *Winnie the Pooh*, leaping up and out and landing right in front of me.

"*Paolamia!*" His excitement radiated off him and onto me, causing my eyes to well up with tears. Papà wrapped his strong arms around me and squeezed tight. In his broken English, he exclaimed: "My baby girl! Papà miss you!"

I did miss my papà. But I missed my new life back at school even more. And I hated myself even more than that for feeling the way I did.

After ushering me into the house, Papà wrestled my luggage into the small landing just inside the front door. He took a step onto the first stair leading up to the living room, kitchen, and bedrooms, allowing me enough space to fully enter. I could see from where I stood that just a few steps to the right there was a downstairs, too.

"Hey, Pauley," Viny called out from above. I looked up, turning my eyes toward her voice. She was kneeling on the couch in the living room that was set against the staircase and the top half of her was hanging over the banister. She waved at me with both hands, giggling with joy.

"Hey, Vince," I smiled back. "I thought you'd still be at Aunt Rose and Uncle Sam's."

"They let me out early for good behavior." Viny exaggerated her laugh.

I laughed in response. "It's not like you were in prison."

"Oh, no?"

As Papà and I climbed the half-dozen or so stairs to the top level, I could see the living room, dining room, and kitchen to the right. Mamma suddenly appeared from the darkened hallway to my left—one that led to the bedrooms, I presumed. When she came into full view, I had to admit, she looked more alive than when I had left her back in August. Her hair didn't seem so tightly wound and the increasing salt in her pepper seemed to shine a bit. Even her lips seemed happier and back to bearing her signature red lipstick—which I assumed she had put on just for my homecoming. Rosario had said she was no longer threatening harm to the family with a house fire, so maybe she really was on the mend?

Hello? Have you met Mamma?

There is no "mend" for schizophrenia. It's not like she's got some broken bone in a cast.

This, too, shall pass. You had your hopes up before.

Don't forget we're dealing with crazy.

Right. But my heart couldn't help but look at her and imagine otherwise.

"Paola!" Mamma's delayed greeting matched her stiff, snail-paced, jerky movements. I stepped closer to her on the landing and hugged her. I regretted inhaling as I did so. While Mamma had tried to mask her bad body odor with Tabu, her favorite perfume, it had only served to make her scent worse.

The doctors blamed it on her body's reaction to the medications. Those cocktails they kept mixing caused side effects that rivaled the actual disorder they were meant to alleviate. I sometimes would have opted for a less catatonic, more schizophrenic Mamma. That said, I definitely would have opted for a more pleasant-smelling Mamma than what I had now. The medications were causing her body to excrete fat. It was as if she was melting, and some sort of yellowish-orange goo on her skin remained as residue. Papà had taken to bathing her, especially since her zombie-like state and Parkinson's-like motor skills had caused her to start neglecting her personal hygiene.

Fats smelled. Badly.

I wondered how Papà could do it. I wondered why he didn't just lock her away permanently. How could he sit on the edge of the tub as she sat in the bath, talking to her softly and scrubbing her back, trying to get that substance off of her? How could he sleep next to Mamma in her condition? Was this what "'til death do us part" included? Count me out. I just couldn't do it for my spouse. I wasn't even sure I could do it for a child.

Mamma clung onto me for longer than I would have liked. "*Aiutami*," she whispered into my ear.

We broke apart. What did she want me to help her with? Her frightened eyes pleaded, betraying her plastered-on smile.

See? Nothing's changed.

Probably not, I surmised, sadly agreeing with the naysayers in my head. But that didn't mean I didn't still care or hope, no matter how much I tried to steel myself against such emotions. I really did wish I could do as Mamma asked. I wanted to help her. I just didn't know how. And it was clear: nobody did.

Papà and I exchanged glances as he slipped past Mamma and me to carry my bags in.

"*Ti piace la nuova casa, Mamma?*" I asked.

I thought to distract her from her call for help by asking her if she liked the new house. Her response—an eerie smile and open-handed palm pump to the heavens—left me a bit unnerved. I had no idea what those gestures meant, and feared the possibilities. Was Rosario wrong? Did she still plan on torching us while we slept?

Mamma slowly turned and carefully walked back down the hallway, returning to the room from whence she'd come. *"Mi vado a fare un sonetto,"* she announced.

As Mamma left to take a nap, Papà returned and excitedly asked me what I thought of the new house. I barely had time to open my mouth to answer when it became clear he didn't really care to know. He immediately launched into an old but familiar topic: Mamma's health.

As he talked about some new drug combination the doctors had given her, I struggled not to glaze over. It wasn't that I didn't care; rather, I had heard it all before and had lost faith in much of anything being able to make a difference.

Papà continued his chatter, telling me about how much he wanted to retire; he was already sixty-eight years old. Thanks to Rosario finding this Algonquin home for $77,500, Papà had been able to pocket about $35,000 from the sale. That kind of money had never been seen before in his bank account. His weekly take-home pay from the last place he'd worked—Fearn International, a food processing plant that made yummy canned soups under the label LeGoût—had totaled $374.50 after taxes. No wonder he seemed so giddy. The very thing he wanted to do—retire—was in sight. Papà was one step closer to being able to live a life of freedom. But he still needed to clear up some of his credit card debt, and, well, figure out how to finance Mamma's illness. If he couldn't figure out how to get her medical bills reduced to some manageable level, he'd never be able to do what he always dreamt of doing.

I barely listened to what Papà was saying. I knew my role of *consigliere* well. Just tell me what we needed to get done, and I was on it. It was my fate, but one I no longer could stomach. I surveyed the upstairs of the home I had yet to tour. Still-unpacked boxes were lined up against the wall from the kitchen to the dining room to the living room. I presumed my stuff had to be somewhere in them, but I didn't bother to ask.

It's just three weeks.

I would keep things in perspective.

"Paola, vieni qui."

My papà led me to a seat in the dining room. Of everything we owned, this table and chairs had always seemed a bit too ornate for us, and now especially didn't belong in this barn of a home. That said, I loved its ball-and-claw feet, and the way the table's legs dramatically curved, as if they were sashaying their hips to a Latin rhythm. The intricately carved backs of the chairs were starting to show their age and neglect. A fine layer of dust had gathered in between the latticed slats, and one had started to split. They were too delicate to handle the weight of any one of us, other than Caterina, who never seemed to gain weight no matter how much she ate.

"Dovè Caterina?" I asked my Papà as I sat in the broken chair.

Papà told me she was at work, then settled himself at the head of the table and pulled out a poem he had written. He hadn't thought to share it before now, he explained, his face blushing a bit. But with what I had said in my letters to him about the professor of my writing class, Papà wondered if I could help him get his poem published.

I turned to Viny. "Vince, is my stuff somewhere?"

She shrugged.

I hadn't been on hand to babysit the care and keeping of my own things during the move over Thanksgiving. I silently prayed that all twenty years' worth of my stuff had made it safely into boxes and survived the trip.

"It's a really good poem." Viny brought me back to Papà's request. "You know, I write poems, too. Do you think I could get published?"

I scrunched up my face as I turned toward her, mustering my best look of disgust. It succeeded in getting Viny to slink down into the couch and out of sight. I looked down at what Papà had written and placed before me. The line he scribbled at the very top indicated that he had written this poem three years earlier, when he had celebrated his sixty-fifth birthday.

He had memorized his words, and he spoke them aloud now. As he lyrically flitted from one line to the next, his tone and tenor became operatic. Gesturing now with his hands, as if in a dance, his final two stanzas brought tears to his eyes.

"I dreamed of the pensioner's life, like a bird that flies in the world, to touch what has not yet been touched and to try its deepest pleasures, reaping the fruits of many years worked.

"Unfortunately, I have to abandon the dream. And even if this wasn't what was envisioned, I am content to embrace the affection of my dear wife and my children. I don't think about it too much. It doesn't cause me upset. Do you know what matters in this world? To be loved and to love the family."

As much as I wanted to give Mamma her freedom from the demons that controlled her, I wanted even more to be able to give Papà the freedom he longed for. He had sacrificed his own life out of love for his family. I felt shame for focusing on my own selfish desires and heard myself promising to get Papà's poem published, despite the fact that I hadn't a clue how.

Pulling out the white handkerchief he always kept in his pocket, Papà dabbed at his eyes and blew his nose. He then placed another poem in front of me, this one dated September 1985.

As I followed along on the page, Papà again wooed with the melody of his words. English didn't do them justice.

Vorrei mettere tutto in poesia
Dal primo giorno che mi son sposato,
Ma penso che mi perdo per la via
Perché la storia è lunga e ho dimenticato.

"I would like to put everything in a poem: From the first day that I got married, but I think that I would get lost along the way, because the story is long and much I have forgotten."

His eyes glistened as he recounted in poetic rhyme how it had been ten years of suffering for Mamma and the family. Leaving one specialist and seeking out another, trying to find the solution that would liberate her from her illness and her tears.

My own heart ached for the pain he poured out, and for his questioning of God—who, I had to agree, seemed to have abandoned us.

Da 10 anni mia Moglie e la Famiglia
2 *soffriamo senza interruzione*
bussiando un Specialista e un'altro piglia
Sperando che mia Moglie si Migliori.

Purtroppo continuano i malanni
3 *Agravando sempre più la situazione*
Il morbo che la sotterra da molti anni
credo che ha fatto annoiare anche ai dottori.

Intanto mia Moglie soffre e soffre tanto
4 *Io non so più che potrei fare*
Per poterla davvero liberare
Dal Suo grande Male e dal Suo pianto.

Spero di non perdere la testa
5 *Nel condurre la mia barca in alto mare*
Qualunque Capitano nel mar in tempesta
Si sarebbe chiesto: devo continuare?

"*I hope not to lose my head in navigating my boat on the high seas. Any captain in such storms would be asking himself: Do I have to continue?*"

Papà's question was the same as mine: Did we have to keep combatting Mamma's illness? When would the madness ever stop? Why couldn't we just be a normal family?

> "*I believe myself to be a good captain, and, therefore, an excellent helmsman. I can maneuver where the waters are calm as well as among hidden reefs and canyons.*"

Papà closed with an impassioned plea to God:

> "*Are we such terrible people to deserve such never-ending pain? Please come and help save my family.*"

It struck me how Papà could still ask something of God that, clearly, God hadn't the power to give or, even worse, had explicitly *chosen* not to give. Just like Job in the Bible, Papà was a man of faith. True, he didn't attend mass every Sunday, but he and Mamma both prayed daily. Furthermore, we always shared what little we had with others. It felt as if this was another example of God wielding his power—taking up a challenge from Satan to prove his people would still worship him even if he made their lives hell on earth for no reason.

I hated the Book of Job, and hated it even more given that we were living a similar story. How much worse could it get? God had killed Job's entire family. Was that what it would come to for us? How could I be grateful for the madness we had been thrust into? It just wasn't fair.

And yet it was exactly where we found ourselves.

CHAPTER SIX: **CAPPELLETTI**

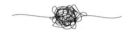

I ENVIED MY FRIENDS DURING this season. Each one seemed to have their own holiday traditions, like one friend who, with her entire family—which included four sisters and one brother— made it their annual Christmas pilgrimage to State Street in the heart of Chicago's downtown. They'd go see the magical displays in department store windows. Then they'd all go to lunch at the famed Marshall Field's Walnut Room. I imagined them, along with hundreds of other families, all dressed up in red, green, and gold seasonal sparkle, sitting in the opulent ballroom under that gorgeously decorated forty-five-foot Christmas tree, eating lunch, sharing stories, and laughing.

We had our own Christmas traditions, too. But more often than not, they included lots of yelling and mostly centered on food.

My sister Caterina accurately explained it as, "Other families plan what they're going to *do* for the holidays. We plan what we're going to *eat*."

I saw nothing wrong with that. It was how we celebrated. As a matter of fact, *not* talking food and menu for the holidays was an indication that something was wrong. Coming home for Christmas, I'd counted on getting to eat some traditional dishes, one of which was called *cappelletti*. These stuffed pasta pockets of chicken and cheese took Mamma and Papà days to make.

They required the duo to manually grind breasts of chicken, grate whole blocks of Pecorino Romano cheese, buy pounds of fresh ricotta, and hand-craft mounds of homemade dough into sheets of pasta to be formed into shapes resembling "little hats"—the English translation of the word *cappelletti*—and stuffed with the scrumptious concoction. I so loved this dish that I often snuck a few of the stuffed pasta pillows from the freezer and ate them raw.

Another Christmas tradition was Mamma's cookies, called *cuccidati*. In truth, I never much cared for these Sicilian fig cookies. I loved Mamma's cookie dough, however, and how the mixture of figs, raisins, nuts, and wine that had been cooked down to a thick, sweet reduction made it taste; I just didn't so much love the actual fig filling.

The best part of these cookies was watching Mamma and Papà working together for days to build them. The smell of the *vino cotto* simmering on the stove, the sounds of that ancient hand-cranked grinder squeaking as it turned to mesh all the ingredients together, the good-natured ribbing between the two of them on how to tweak the recipe "next time" for added flavor—*that*, to me, was Christmas.

Only "next time," which was this particular Christmas, included none of what I knew home for the holidays to be. No *cappelletti*. No *cuccidati*. No Mamma and Papà working together in the kitchen. Not this Christmas. *Buon Natale* seemed to be on leave this year.

Caterina tried to make the best of it. She had sent me letters weeks prior while I was still at ISU, telling me that we'd go Christmas shopping together when I got home, and that she had already bought part of my gift. She was trying to do the big sister thing to cheer me, and herself, up. I don't think it was working for either of us.

I had my own role to play as big sister to Viny, knowing she had to get out of that house and be around people. Her isolation, I could tell, was weakening her mind and spirit further. She was spending more time than ever before locked away on her own. It wasn't healthy.

My human GPS was bad enough when I knew where I was, but here in the middle of new surroundings, it was even worse. There had to be services for people like Viny. But where? And how? And what could I really set up for her in just these couple of weeks while on break when everybody else seemed to be on break too?

As it turned out, I found a lot. The county we had moved into, McHenry County, had recently expanded its vocational rehabilitation services for people with disabilities, both mental and developmental. Not only would Viny be eligible to participate in social activities in their day programs but they would send out a van to pick her up each morning and to bring her home.

Viny wasn't thrilled about the idea; in fact, she repeatedly dismissed it.

As I slept on the living room couch—the only place there was for me to sleep, I tossed and turned, wondering if it was or wasn't the right thing to do for her. What other choices were there?

Since I couldn't seem to fall asleep, I mulled over the pros and cons, waiting for the winter sun to rise. The street light at the corner of our lot seemed determined to shine in my eyes no matter where I put my head. I figured I should just get up and make something for breakfast when all of a sudden, coming from the other room, I heard a loud rustling, followed by a thud, followed by an expletive of, "*Gesu!*"

My papà's whispers to Mamma sounded so panicked. "*Maria, dove sono le mie calzette?*"

Mamma's faint voice responded back with where his socks were, as dresser drawers opened and slammed shut.

I looked at the clock. 5:00 a.m.? Papà was usually out the door by this time. I hunkered back down underneath my covers as their old bed creaked loudly. I imagined Papà had found his socks and was pulling them on.

It took a good hour to get from Algonquin to Franklin Park, where Papà worked at Fearn International. He needed to clock in by 6:00 a.m. or get his pay docked—or worse. We couldn't afford worse.

Mamma's voice whispered more loudly, "*Subito, subito!*"

Yeah, I thought to myself: *Hurry!*

As Papà made his way out of his bedroom and down the hall, not even stopping to go to the bathroom, it was clear to me from all the thumping around that he was knocking into the walls, probably still half asleep. I listened as his footsteps pounded down each stair from our living room to the downstairs recreation room, then out the door and into the garage.

In the short time I had been home, I already had gotten used to the grinding of the electric door opening and shutting. This morning, however, I heard that door start to open and then stop seconds later. It happened again. The door gears kept getting started and then just stopping. On the third try, and with Papà's frustrated cry of, "*Porca miseria!*" reaching my ears, the door finally rose all the way to the top. Finally, I heard the roar of our silver Pontiac's engine turning over, the revving of my papà's foot pushing on the gas, and the car pulling away and onto the street. The sound of the garage door shutting never came. I figured Papà had left it open, either forgetting to shut it or out of frustration not wanting to chance it refusing to come down.

As I rose to make coffee, heading first downstairs to close the garage door, I hoped Papà would make it to work without any more issues. He would be turning sixty-nine in March. That was too old for anybody to still be working—especially if, like Papà, the work was manual.

LATER THAT NIGHT, I HAD just finished watching *The Jeffersons* with Viny, and we were both belting out the lyrics of the theme song—Viny knew the lyrics of every song, or so it seemed, and her voice was totally on pitch, too; she had inherited Papà's vocals for sure—when the sound of the garage door rising prompted us to scramble downstairs to greet Papà. Mamma joined us, too. I think we all were a bit worried about his late start that day and even Mamma wanted to make sure he was okay.

We waited just inside the door for him to turn off the engine and step out of the driver's seat. Before we could actually see him, we heard his voice telling us there were groceries in the trunk for us to help bring inside.

As we walked into the garage and over to the back end of the car, Papà met us there.

"*Ma che cosa?*" Mamma started to laugh, with one hand covering her mouth and the other pointing to Papà's head.

Viny and I howled when we saw what had Mamma giggling. Our almost bald Papà was wearing a poofy shower cap on his head. He was required to wear a hairnet to work in the food processing plant, but we had never actually seen what he looked like with one on. The very ridiculousness of someone bald wearing a hairnet, let alone one that looked as big as that, had us all doubled over.

"*Dio santo!*" Papà let out, and started laughing louder than us all. In between his chuckling, he confessed that he had been wondering why everyone in the grocery store kept staring at him and trying not to laugh. He then slapped his forehead and tossed back his head, roaring, sharing that he had even stopped to pump gas with it on!

We each wiped away tears of laughter as we grabbed bags of groceries and carried them upstairs into the kitchen. After putting them away, we all sat down to dinner. Rosario and Caterina were both at work.

I had twirled a forkful of spaghetti and was directing it into my mouth when I happened to look down and noticed my papà's socks. One was white, and the other was black. I had to put my fork down as I burst out laughing for the second time that day.

When I was able to spit out what had me in stitches, Papà just shook his head, chuckling as he put down his own fork to tell us about the rest of his day. He began talking with his hands, bestowing yet another Sicilian proverb as a lesson to us all.

"*Cui lassa la via vecchia pri la nova, li guai ch'un va circannu, ddà li trova,*" he laughingly said—"He who leaves the old road for the new will often find himself in trouble."

Papà had had a little brush with the law that morning. He had thought to take a new route to work, one that might be faster since he was so late. He turned down Route 72 and gave thanks that no one else seemed to be on the road. Pushing the speed limit a bit, he suddenly saw the red and blue flashing lights in his rearview mirror. He knew he wasn't going so fast as to warrant a ticket; maybe they weren't coming after him, he told us he thought. He slowly swerved to the side to let the officers pass him by, but they didn't. Instead, two of the squad cars flanked him on both sides while the third stayed directly behind him.

While he tried to think through every move he had made since leaving the house that morning, he couldn't come up with a single reason for them to come after him. Finally, he slowed the car to a stop in the staging lane to the right of the highway. He rolled down his window and waited.

When all three of the officers came up to his driver's side, Papà admitted to us that he was a bit scared. He nervously asked them in his best broken English, *"Excuzami Ufficiale.* Maybe I make mistake?"

The younger officer asked to see his driver's license, which Papà quickly handed over.

The second officer asked, "Where are you going?"

Papà tsked and answered, "I be late for work. *Mia famiglia* move here couple weeks before, and I take this road 72 first time."

The third and eldest of the officers smiled and let out a chuckle. "Well you're never going to get anywhere from here. This is Route 72 alright, but it's one-way, and you're going the wrong way."

"No!" Papà said he put both his hands on his head.

"Tell you what," the older officer said as the younger one handed him back his license. "Where do you work?"

"Franklin Park."

"What time do you start?"

"Six o'clock."

Papà told us it was already about 5:30 a.m. when he got stopped, and it usually took another forty minutes to get to work from where they had stopped him.

"Let's get you back on the road. You follow me, *capisce?*" The older cop winked and jogged over to his squad car. With his red and blue lights still flashing, he drove out in front of Papà at well over the speed limit. When they crossed the boundaries into Franklin Park, the officer turned off his lights and waved good-bye to Papà.

At this point, Papà's laughter had a tinge of sorrow. His eyes glassed over, glistening. He nodded as he told us he made it to work with two minutes to spare.

"*Un miracolo,*" Mamma said, making the sign of the cross.

Papà agreed that it was a miracle.

THAT NIGHT, WE ALL FELT pretty grateful. And Mamma felt well enough to keep with tradition by making us *Sfingi.* These Sicilian donuts were one of her specialties, another treat that she only made once a year. The sound of her beating the dough with her right hand and the smell of the yeasty-yumminess frying in oil, then her rolling them in sugar while they were still warm were reason to get excited . . . and loosen our pants. We ate and ate and ate, laughing about Papà and his crazy day, as if we were normal.

ON CHRISTMAS DAY, AS WAS our tradition, we all piled into Papà's silver Pontiac and headed off to morning mass. As cafeteria Catholics, Christmas and Easter were the two days we made an appearance. Just being back at St. Lambert's Church, however, made my insides churn.

I couldn't help but think of that Christmas so long ago, back when I was in the eighth grade, when Mamma, who after a couple of years of refusing, had decided to join us for Christmas Day services. What Papà had thought was a miracle—Mamma feeling well enough to come along—I'd known had to be something else. And I'd ended up being right.

During communion, Mamma had thrown herself at our parish priest's feet, her screams bouncing off the stained glass windows and echoing throughout the halls as she begged for someone to save her from her family—which, she said, was trying to kill her.

Up until that point, no one outside the family had known of Mamma's mental illness. But at that moment, our secret had been exposed to the entire congregation, including friends and teachers.

Now back in that same church, I held my breath during the entire service, waiting and wondering when the next shoe would drop. But it never did. The entire Christmas break at home, while not exactly celebratory, was not a disaster. At least, not the one I had dreaded it would be.

It actually proved to be pretty calm. Crazy must have needed a holiday—at least, I hoped that was its reason. As much as things seemed almost stable, I wondered if it was all pretend. Crazy often kept itself hidden, secretly growing, preparing for its next move and moment to pounce. I always tried to stay on guard.

Nothing to see here.

For now.

CHAPTER SEVEN: **CHARACTER**

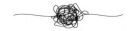

SOON, I FOUND MYSELF BACK in my dorm at ISU. Beth and Kathy had already arrived. We shared quick recaps of our holidays at our respective homes. I, of course, got creative with my experiences.

You mean you lied.

They were only white lies, I argued back. And really, it was more for their benefit than mine. They wanted to know what Christmas in the big city of Chicago was like. So I told them. I never said it was *my* Christmas experience.

Liar.

I had gotten good at lying. I never really meant to be untruthful or misleading; it just came naturally, sometimes for self-preservation and sometimes to give myself permission to pretend that what I wished for was, indeed, reality. There was so much about me and my life that wasn't normal: my family's Sicilian code of keeping whatever happened in the family secret from the outside world; Mamma's schizophrenic mind and her thoughts that we were trying to kill her or that I was some kind of sexual deviant; Viny's failure to thrive academically, socially, and physically; and, speaking of physically, my own ever-growing size. I now tipped the scales at 250 pounds no matter what I tried to do to lose weight.

Liar. You mean no matter how you pretend *to try and lose weight.*

Okay, I *was* pretending. I just no longer seemed to care enough to even try. I'd never be skinny. It just wasn't in my genes. Maybe my family's insanity genes had swapped places with my skinny genes. I laughed at the thought of it.

SO ON THAT DAY BACK AT SCHOOL, when the new teacher bounded into the room like a Mack truck barreling downhill, not bothering to even tap on the brakes, I paid attention.

"Defamation, privacy, copyright, obscenity, the lottery, the FCC, advertising, the press . . . Welcome to Journalism Mass Communication 460. I'm Professor Barbara Mack."

She was big. She was loud. She was intimidating. And she was totally in control. From the moment she started speaking, she barely let up to take a breath.

Neither did I, I realized; I was holding my breath during her entire introduction. I also realized that I'd loved her from the moment she entered the room.

How tall she actually was, I couldn't guess. But even without the black pumps she wore, her Amazon-like presence towered and commanded attention. With every move she made, her wavy, shoulder-length, dark brown hair bounced like a Breck girl's. Dressed in a gray wool pantsuit over a bright blue blouse with a single strand of pearls, she looked as if she belonged more in a courtroom than a classroom.

"If you didn't intend to take this media law class, then I suggest you pick up your things and leave now, before we get started," she said as she settled her purse that looked more like a briefcase, armfuls of papers and books, and all else she was carrying on the top of her desk. She then leaned back against her desk to look at us all, flashing a smile that seemed to be trying not to erupt into full-on laughter.

This was the first classroom I was in at ISU where the setup wasn't auditorium or lecture style, with a bunch of seats in rows and columns facing front. Instead, we were all seated at the same continuous tables, arranged to form a U-shape. I couldn't have been more grateful. I hated trying to focus on the teacher at the front of the room while trying to navigate around an obstructed view, courtesy of some melon-headed kid who always seemed to be seated directly in front of me. Being squished in between the other twenty or more students gathered as Dr. Mack held court should have made me uncomfortable, but I didn't mind one bit. I barely even noticed anyone else in the room, once I set eyes on her.

Dr. Mack began telling us "a little bit" about herself.

She'd started out as a news assistant and then a reporter for the *Des Moines Register & Tribune*. She'd earned her bachelor's degree in journalism from Iowa State and gotten her juris doctorate from Drake University. This was her first year as a faculty member at ISU, which for us, she joked, could be a good thing or very, very bad.

Her throaty laugh boomed as she threw back her head. She so reminded me of Kathleen Turner's character in the 1981 film *Body Heat*. With every line she delivered, she effortlessly shifted from hardcore disciplinarian judge and jury to fun-filled, mischievous entertainer laced with just the right amount of caregiving mom. All I could think was, *I want to be like you when I grow up.*

On that first day of class, Dr. Mack started out with what she said was an easy, open-and-shut kind of situation.

"It's the same as if—let's say—I had agreed to purchase your heifer, and three months later, she were to miraculously give birth to a calf." Dr. Mack waved her hands in the air, then pointed her fingers my way. "Tell me, what legal rights might you be entitled to?"

I froze. My mind raced. I wanted to speak, but nothing would come out. Dr. Mack cocked an eyebrow, and all the other students seemed to lean forward in anticipation.

Sputtering a bit, I finally squeaked out a response: "Um . . . sorry, Dr. Mack, but what's a heifer?"

The room immediately howled with laughter, Professor Mack perhaps the loudest among them. All eyes were on me, including those of a girl sitting directly across from me on the opposite side of the U-shaped desks. Her chortle was more of a Santa-like ho-ho-ho, but when she caught my eye, her expression immediately switched to a poker face.

"You're not from around here, are you?" Professor Mack quipped, giving me a wink as she struggled to stop laughing.

"Chicago," I said.

Dr. Mack nodded, working her way into the center of the desks' U. "Well, Chicago, a heifer is, in essence, a virgin cow. So can you see the dilemma if that's what you paid for, but a few months down the road, she's giving birth?"

I nodded, and Dr. Mack moved on. I wanted to disappear. While the students redirected their attentions to Dr. Mack's lesson, I could feel my cheeks still flushed from embarrassment.

A virgin cow. How ironic.

Reminded of my sexual status and physical appearance all at once, I shut down—lowered my gaze and tuned out the lively conversation that had ensued.

A voice rang out, I assumed in response to what was being discussed. Suddenly, I heard the words "city girl" and looked up, bracing myself to be the butt of a joke. The girl I had made eye contact with moments before was speaking.

"I know what a heifer is," she said, "but I'm not planning on sticking around here after I graduate."

"Your point being?" Dr. Mack cocked one eyebrow.

"Are there examples that aren't about farm life?" As much as the second part of what she said sounded less confident, the girl still said it. And I felt she said it in defense of me.

Who is that?

We like her.

I couldn't be sure. But why would she even bother to say something if it wasn't in response to everybody laughing at me? I felt a little bit like that kid in that 1980s coming-of-age movie *My Bodyguard.* I wasn't getting bullied like he was, and I hadn't hired this classmate to be my bodyguard like he had, but, oddly, it felt the same. It was as if she had decided to take on that role of protector. I only wondered why, and what it would end up costing me in the end. If there was one thing I had learned in my life, it was that everything came with a price.

The girl and I exchanged glances. She seemed so sure of herself, underscoring what she had just said with a nod of her head. It was only then that I noticed her size. She was as full-figured as I was, maybe even more.

Why didn't we notice her earlier?

Professor Mack nodded and said that from now on, she would use examples referencing things that "the rest of the world" worked with; heifers and farm life were, indeed, not all there was. Suddenly, I was back to being just another normal nobody. Fellow students ignored me when class was over. It no longer mattered what I had said, except to the girl who had chimed in on my behalf.

"You are *hilarious!*" She said to me in a deep, husky voice as we exited Dr. Mack's class. The girl's round face and blue eyes reminded me of the famous Gerber baby: this was what she'd look like all grown up.

"I am?" I said, not really meaning to use my outside voice.

She nodded, all smiles, and then held out her hand in an official kind of way. "I'm Shelly. Michelle, actually, but my friends call me Shelly."

I decided to use my Americanized name instead of my real Sicilian one. It just seemed to fit better on a farm. "Paula." I nodded back and extended my hand to shake hers.

Shelly and I headed out in the same general direction.

At a full six feet tall, Shelly seemed to tower over me. We shared the same plus-size body type and even the same long, dark, curly hair. Shelly, however, had clearly mastered the art of face painting; her makeup was applied just so. My face remained a blank canvas. Mamma had slapped me when I was young for even trying a little eye shadow, considering it to be the stuff whores wore. So I'd just never taken to the stuff. Certainly not like Shelly.

Or any other normal girl your age.

I quickly learned two things about this girl: She already had turned twenty-one the year prior, whereas I would turn of legal drinking age in about a month; and she had already had sex, more than once and with more than one person, whereas I had yet to be asked to hook up, let alone consent to it.

While I had always assumed my lack of popularity with the boys was due to my weight, hanging out with Shelly made me question my beliefs. When I shared with Shelly how I thought everybody was looking at me because I was fat, she shared that she was confident that everybody was looking at her because she was so hot.

Shelly was a local, blue collar farm girl who ran a bit on the wild side and lived life as if every moment was her last, with no apologies or regrets—at least that's how I viewed her. I, on the other hand, was always responsible and forever felt guilty (warranted or not) about anything and everything, especially sex (whether I was having it or was assumed to be having it—which, did I mention I was not?)—a casualty of my being first-generation Sicilian and raised to be a "good Catholic girl."

In many ways, I envied my new friend.

As opposite as we were alike, we instantly connected.

Shelly was drawn to my big-city status. While it was true that I was born in Chicago, I had been raised in a much sleepier suburb of Skokie, far from the skyscrapers, nightclubs, and bright lights Shelly seemed to think I frequented—but I didn't correct her. I let her think I was much cooler than she'd soon figure me out to be.

Our points of differentiation really came into focus when it came to sex. It wasn't that Shelly was promiscuous; rather, it was just that she really, really, really loved sex. And she made it normal for me to want to have it too.

I wondered what Mamma would have done to Shelly if she had been her daughter. I had been raised to believe that only bad girls had sex before marriage, yet Shelly seemed to be on a mission to educate me and any other girl interested on why it was bad for anyone to wait to have sex until they were married. Just a few of her thoughts for consideration included: *Why would you want to have sex with just one partner your whole life? What if he doesn't know a G spot from a G string? What about his size, or making sure that if he isn't big, he knows how to do other things, or at least how to move?* Or, as she put it: *It's not the size of the ocean but the motion of the wave. What if there isn't any chemistry between the two of you?*

Shelly made valid arguments. Dr. Mack would have been proud. And I would have paid more attention if, indeed, I was purposely saving myself for marriage. But I wasn't. I just didn't have anybody who was interested.

For me, Shelly brought to life everything I never knew existed: she was the first big, beautiful, confident, sexy girl I had ever encountered. And Dr. Mack was equally as big and confident and beautiful, with a lot more wisdom to boot.

It was clear that Dr. Mack shared Shelly's enthusiasm for sex. While usually punctual for class, one morning, she kept us all waiting in our seats. It was pretty typical for students to leave if a professor didn't show up after the first ten minutes, but nobody wanted to miss one of Dr. Mack's classes, so we all stayed. When she finally did show up, she flew into class, her hair messed up, her face flushed, and one breast threatening to pop out of her blouse, which had clearly been hurriedly tossed on, given the mismatched buttoning.

I raised my eyebrows, as I'm sure we all did. I may have even let out a tiny gasp. Dr. Mack was always so put together, yet here she was, definitely *not*. When I looked at Shelly, she had such a knowing grin on her face. I could tell she was doing all she could not to belt out laughing.

"Well!" Dr. Mack paused to let out a breath, dropped her briefcase onto the top of her desk, and swung her hair back and forth, smoothing it down with her two hands. It wasn't until then that she realized she was pretty much exposing herself, just a tiny bit.

The moment she noticed, she erupted in a brassy laugh, turned her back to us, and adjusted her blouse.

"What can I say?" she cheerfully sang out, spinning herself back to face us moments later. "My husband Jim's home early."

For the rest of that day and for days to come, Shelly and I couldn't stop laughing about Dr. Mack and her early-morning-wake-up-call-induced wardrobe malfunction. We also talked a lot about finding "the one"—the guy who would mess up your hair, undo your buttons, make you late for class, and marry you so you could live together happily ever after.

Is there really such a thing?

Doubtful.

Even my college-degreed, loved-to-dance sister Caterina, with her perfect body and pretty face, struggled back home to find her own forever guy. And Papà had thought Mamma was his perfect person; he even still did, in a way, though that feeling was now dampened with her illness. Even Rosario seemed to doubt the wisdom of committing himself to any one person. He loved to quote Zsa Zsa Gabor, who said, "A man is not complete until he is married. Then, he is finished."

I found myself with more and more evidence to support the possibility that there really was no happily ever after. Could you only get that blissful happiness Dr. Mack seemed to possess from finding someone to love? Shelly seemed happy. She didn't have anybody special. Was the key to being happy falling in love with yourself first?

I hadn't any answers.

JUST AS I WAS SETTLING BACK into my life at ISU, I suddenly found myself with even more questions, thanks to the stream of letters from home that once again resumed.

Caterina's letter arrived just about a week after spring semester started. She wrote on a Sunday night, saying that she dreaded her Monday morning return to work. She said she envied people who knew their true calling. She wanted to do something meaningful in her life, but ever since finishing school, she was so confused about what that might be and wasn't finding meaning in anything she was currently doing.

keep thinking I have to do something more meaningful with my life. Only I don't know what. I envy those people who know their "calling." All I do know, is that I really have to get off my royal duff & start searching. Ever since I finished School, I am so confused I can't find meaning in virtually anything I do.

She'd crossed out "virtually": That bothered me. She found no meaning in *anything*? Would I feel the same way she did after my own graduation? Would I even get to graduate? What was *my* true calling? What if I never found it?

ISU'S OUTSTANDING BILLS SAT next to me on my bed. They remained unopened. I already knew what they had to communicate, I could almost recite it by heart: Each term, students who did not pay their first payment in full by the due date would automatically be charged a $20 administrative fee. University fees were due for spring semester just after Valentine's Day. Grades would be withheld until all fees were paid in full.

I was beginning to realize the consistent themes appearing in my life: money, dieting, and mental illness—not always in that order.

Viny's latest letter did bring a smile to my face, as much as it also pained me to read her words. Her sense of humor and efforts at her penmanship came through clearly. I couldn't recall ever having seen her words so carefully written, painstakingly staying within the ruled lines of the notebook paper. Her comedic perspective on dieting had me envisioning her with a babushka scarf wrapped around her head, attempting her best Russian accent, performing her own little skit—to an empty room, sadly.

"Hey" Did you notice I'm starting off with Hey like Mallory's boyfriend The other way is formal are you getting fat like me I hope not I'm starting to look like a slob or a Russian woman with hairy under arms now I'm trying to diet forget about that stupid subject on oprah's show They had 2nd grade boys doing the shuffle.

bye   love Vincenza

My little sister's cognitive growth, or lack thereof, showed itself plainly in her writing, if anyone was bothering to pay attention. Misspellings of simple words, missing punctuation, and the jumbled way she communicated her thoughts further underscored the fact that my nineteen-year-old sister had stalled in grammar school and possessed the intelligence and emotional equivalency of, at best, a seventh or eighth grader, someone around the age of twelve. Being in such close quarters with her during Christmas break served as another reminder of her solitary existence and that she was only falling further and further behind. That was why I'd pushed so hard while at home to get her enrolled in some outside social services.

Viny never spelled her name the same, I had noticed with her signatures in her letters. "Vincenzina" was her given name. In Italian, it's beautiful. In English, it's a challenge. Teachers called her "Viny" and then sometimes would spell it with one "n" and sometimes with two. Here Viny had written her name as "Vincenza," so either she was testing out yet another version of herself, or perhaps she'd just run out of room on the paper and was trying to be neat.

Learning from what she had written in her letter, I was grateful she had started watching *Oprah*. Maybe she would find herself in that TV show. The fact she even referenced the subject of dieting was a good sign, too. At least with Oprah, she might not feel so alone.

It was the same with me and Shelly and Dr. Mack. I felt that if these two bigger-than-life women were succeeding on their own terms, maybe I could, too.

Papà's letter elicited within me the same reaction Viny's had. His side note, what he had scribbled in the margin to the left, made me chuckle: He had lost ten pounds! I didn't even know Papà cared about his weight. He must have been watching *Oprah*, too!

"*Tutto normale*," he had written. "Everything's normal."

I wondered if I was the only one in our family who understood just how *not* normal everything actually was. It wasn't normal for Mamma to hear voices and to see visions and to believe her family was trying to kill her. It wasn't normal for Viny to have her mental and physical deficiencies go mostly unnoticed, for her needs to continuously fall through the cracks. It wasn't normal for my older sister to be smart and pretty, yet not where she deserved to be in her professional or personal life. We were anything but normal.

Or is this what normal really means?

I refused to believe this was it, the best it would be.

I read further: Papà confirmed that the McHenry County Social Services I had registered Viny to begin attending, a program at something they called Pioneer Center, had actually started. This good news offered me the tiniest bit of comfort. I gave thanks that Viny was eligible for services, including vocational training and socialization among her peers. If nothing else, I prayed that Viny might find a friend and a possible path toward a job at which she could earn a little money and feel a sense of accomplishment and success. Nineteen years was a long time to feel so alone and like a complete failure.

No way was that normal.

> Vincenzina lunedì 27 gennaio, incomincia a frequentare quell'Istituto.
> Una Ven, la mattina alle ore otto viene a casa nostra e la porta in quello Istituto e la riportano a casa verso le 3 del pomeriggio.
> Vincenzina pare che ci va contenta; speriamo si riuscirà a qualche cosa.

The final bit of this letter from home included Mamma's message to me. I could tell by her handwriting and what she shared that at the moment she took pen to paper, her voices were silent and her delusions had disappeared. For now.

> *"Ti penso sempre e ti dico che tutti noi sentiamo la mancanza di te."*

It took a lot for Mamma to express her feelings. For her to write that she thought of me always and that everyone missed me reminded me of the Mamma she wanted to be, the one who was present when her demons weren't.

". . . auguro che l'anno che viene la sculoa la farai a Chicago così stiamo vicino come prima."

She hoped that the following year, I would continue my schooling in Chicago, so that we could be close like we were before.

Her desire to have me near and to, most likely, comfort me with that thought resulted in the very opposite feeling within me. My inevitable return to what wasn't normal for anybody other than me and my family sent tremors throughout my body—tremors that, for me, could be soothed only by the consumption of mass quantities of food.

PROFESSOR HADLEY—OR LEE, as we all called her by now—burst into the classroom like a ray of sunshine pushing its way out of a gray, frothy bunch of clouds. She barely waited to reach the front of the room before sharing what had her so excited.

"Our next assignment!" She nearly shouted it out to us.

Since we had all recently been away for Christmas break, Lee announced, she wanted us to give her a glimpse into our respective worlds by putting it down in a story.

Are you kidding?

I totally echoed the same sentiments.

"Glimpses of . . . whatever you want to share," Lee explained. The example she offered up was something called *Glimpses of Academia*. She handed out copies, several pages, double-spaced, by someone none of us knew. It featured snippets of scantron sheets with their rows of bubbles blackened in alongside digestible bites of story that told of what life was like in the world of education from that writer's perspective. That was what Lee wanted from us.

This is bad.

I agreed. No good could come from sharing with Lee and the rest of the class what my world back at home was like. Until now, I had done a good job of keeping crazy at bay while at school.

A great job!

No one at school knew anything about my home life. What little they did know was what I wanted them to believe, what I wished was the truth. Big-city girl, Sicilian family full of food and fun—that was who they knew me to be. And I wanted it to stay that way. I wanted, just for a little while, for everything in my world not to revolve around schizophrenia or around having to take care of everybody else. I wanted to pretend that, just for a little while, my life was about me. I almost stopped picking up my mail. I should have. If it wasn't the letters from home, it was the notices from ISU about late payments due to the school that were stressing me out. I did not have the money, and there wasn't anybody in the family I could ask for it, either.

I had sent a letter to the women I had worked with at the Bridal Registry. In it, I had mentioned to them that just before leaving for school, I had gotten food poisoning at D.B. Kaplan's, and that the restaurant's manager had called and offered me a couple of free meals in exchange for not participating in or pursuing any litigation.

Mrs. Stone, one of the ladies with whom I had worked, was probably the fiercest among them. Tall and lanky, she was the Jewish mom you didn't mess with. She also was the wife of a pretty high-powered attorney in Chicago. They both had encouraged me to sue. I didn't want to—legal fees weren't something I could even think of adding to my debt—but Mrs. Stone insisted, telling me to leave it all with her and her husband. She also said she'd let me know when my "millions" were on their way. Not that I was banking on it, but at this point, I sure hoped she wasn't kidding. I would gratefully settle for a couple of thousand, just enough to pay my bills and get my grades before I headed home.

At that moment, however, there was nothing I could do about my situation, other than pretend it wasn't what it was. I could definitely do that. Besides, if I didn't get going, I would be late to my horseback riding class. So I shoved the letters and all the worries back into my secret shoebox, hid it in its usual place, grabbed my jacket, and headed out the door.

The stables where the horses were kept were nearly one mile one way from my dorm room. Because of my navigational deficiencies, more often than not, I'd end up turned around, doubling the distance and the time it took to get to and from class. No wonder horseback riding was listed under Physical Education in the course catalog: I got a workout before ever getting near a single horse. Actually, when I thought about it, I realized that the class was much more about the care and keeping of these four-legged friends than riding off with them into the sunset, as I had envisioned myself doing.

Class really wasn't a class at all. There weren't any other students, and we didn't meet in a classroom or lecture hall. It was pretty much just me, myself, and I. And of course, my horse, who, ironically, was named Charlie, too. But whereas Charlie the cadaver never moved or got out of line, this Charlie couldn't seem to stand still and was constantly pulling pranks on me.

I'd come into his stall with my bucket of tools—combs, brushes, hoof picks, sponges, sprays—and after I set them down and moved toward his head to secure him with a quick-release knot, he'd purposely start pulling things out of the bucket and tossing them to the ground. The more I told him to knock it off, the more he thought we were playing.

He was lucky he was so handsome. His velvety hazelnut coat shimmered in the sunlight, and his chocolate mane and tail reminded me of some long-haired hero from a Harlequin romance novel. Of course, to get him to his Fabio best, I had to groom him in the way I had been taught.

Running my hand down his leg to pick up his hoof for cleaning, I felt for bumps or scrapes and made sure he didn't have rocks in his hooves. Once that was done, I combed him in a circular motion with one of the brushes, starting at his neck and moving backward toward his rump. Clouds of dust would swirl about, and as much as I was getting him cleaned up, I was getting dirtier with every stroke.

Charlie loved to have his belly brushed. When he was done, he let me know by swinging his head so that it was directly on top of mine and nibbling on my hair.

"Charlie!" I'd push him off of me so that I could finish. As much as this wasn't exactly what I had signed up for, I had to admit, I felt such a connection with this animal. Hours would go by, well beyond the boundaries of class time, and I'd lean into Charlie just as he would lean into me. The smell of springtime and the scent of my horse were intoxicating. I often showed up late to work to care for my other Charlie.

Janet understood, and usually greeted me by asking how Charlie number two was doing.

I just smiled at her, knowing that she had to know the peace I felt when spending time with my horse.

I felt equally connected to life when cleaning out the terrarium on Janet's desktop. I especially loved the little garter snake. I'd take him out of his home first, ahead of the salamander and toad, and let him coil himself in between the fingers of my hand. He loved resting there, and I loved the silky feel of him against my skin.

Only on this particular day, the snake was missing. I called Janet over to help look. Sometimes, the snake and the salamander would hide inside one of the hollow tree branches or under the rock-like structure that Janet had placed inside their glass garden. She found the salamander, who seemed to be hiding, but no snake.

Janet then noticed the toad and his protruding belly.

"Oh my God!" Janet sucked in her breath when she realized the very sad fact that the toad had eaten our snake.

"No way," I said.

"Way!" she spat out angrily, and then, without any discussion, she wrapped herself into her jacket, reached into the container to grab the toad, and took him out of the office.

I continued to care for the salamander, cleaning him and his cage, until Janet returned a few moments later without the toad.

"What did you do?" I asked

"I released him back into the wild," she said clapping her hands together triumphantly. "He clearly knows how to find food."

"But Janet, isn't it too cold outside for him?" I had no idea if it was or wasn't, but if someone my size still needed to wear a jacket at this time of year, how would a little amphibian fare on his own out there?

Janet sat back down on her desk chair with a huff. "He should have thought of that before eating my snake!"

I felt bad for the little guy, and hoped he'd survive outside on his own. Janet did have a point. The toad should have known better than to eat one of his roomies. But then again, did amphibians really think that far out? Did they even think at all? Most humans didn't. And most humans seemed to prey on those not in a position to fight back.

I WAS STILL THINKING ABOUT this when our dorm had its floor party. It was my first.

Beth stood in front of the mirror in our dorm room, brushing her hair. She had met a boy and would be going out with him that night. He had told her that he loved the muscles on her back. I cringed at the thought of any guy touching my back.

He wouldn't find muscles, more like fat rolls.

Exactly.

After Beth left, I intended to stay in my room all night. But outside my door, the noise level was so loud, and I was so curious to see what a college party might be like. So eventually I decided to get dressed and boldly go where I had never gone before. I had no clue why I would have packed a pair of black heels, but I had, and I decided to wear them with my jeans and an oversized sweater.

A boy I was interested in was at the party. I didn't know his name. All I did know was that he came from a town in Iowa called Bettendorf. That's what I called him: "Bettendorf"—the boy with the dark, Sylvester Stallone kind of eyes.

Bettendorf was sharing a drink with one of the other girls on the floor. I didn't know her name either, but I had seen her from time to time, in the bathroom usually. I had dubbed her Mouse. She seemed so small, thin, and frail, always scampering around as if trying to hide from view. Mouse seemed to fit her. I was surprised she was even at the party—or maybe I was just surprised at what looked like a real-life Rocky and Adrian scenario. Could someone like Mouse really attract someone like Bettendorf? She looked sickly, in dire need of getting some sun. Her skin tone was a dingy off-white with a yellowish tint—the kind of color that shows up after bruises start to fade.

I did my best to ignore the two of them and tried to walk to the beat of the music. One of my favorites was playing: The Outfield's "Your Love." I felt all eyes on me as I did my best not to wobble on the high heels I clearly shouldn't have worn.

They're waiting to see how long before you fall on your ass. Or your face.

Panic started to set in and sweat gathered on my upper lip, as I knew very well that the voices' predictions were a very real possibility.

Remember what Shelly said. They're looking at you because you're hot.

Fat chance.

This was a giant mistake. You should have just stayed in your room.

I was handed a red plastic cup with booze in it. I swayed to the music, lip-syncing the words I knew, and looked around for Bettendorf and Mouse. He was still there, now talking to another group of guys, but Mouse had vanished from sight. Another plastic cup replaced the one I had in my hand.

What were you thinking coming here?

You don't belong here.

The music seemed so loud. Another favorite tune: "Tarzan Boy" by Baltimora. I wondered if Rosario had heard of them. I set my drink down on one of the tables against the wall, right next to the kegs of beer. Someone handed me another red plastic cup, and I took it.

People all around me were dancing, laughing, kissing. I stood alone.

Drink in hand, I stumbled down the hall to my dorm room, or what I thought was my room. The door was unlocked. I knew I had locked mine, but that didn't stop me. Pushing my way inside, I froze at the sight of Mouse sitting on the bottom bunk of the bed, her head struggling to free itself from the hand that was clamped over it, trying to push it down, as she tried to keep it up. I blinked a few times before following the hand to its owner: some guy I had never seen before, sitting beside Mouse, and trying to force her head into his crotch area. He still had his pants zipped, but from the bulge that had grown underneath his jeans, it was clear even to me what he intended for Mouse to do, whether or not she was on board.

A few moments later, the boy noticed me standing in the doorway. He immediately released Mouse's head and stood up, as if he and his plans had been found out—which, of course, was exactly what was happening. Brusquely brushing past me, he left the room.

Mouse looked up at me: her eyes could barely focus; her hair was wet and plastered to her forehead. She lifted one hand and waved at me. I nodded, stepped back out into the hallway, and then locked her door from the inside and shut it behind me.

It dawned on me that whatever I was drinking was the same stuff Mouse had been drinking. Clearly, it wasn't what was best for either of us. Partying wasn't for me, and I was okay with returning to my own dorm room, locking my own door, and waiting for the night to come to an end.

CHAPTER EIGHT: **CIRCUSES**

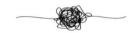

PARTYING WASN'T MY THING. Surprises weren't either. I much preferred controlling whatever happened or was going to happen before it ever had a chance to actually happen.

My upcoming twenty-first birthday was something I didn't want to happen. Expectations came with being legal to drink. Normal college students trolled the bars in celebration. I wasn't normal.

I'd felt the same for my eighteenth birthday. I'd known something was up when driving home from my shift at the Marshall Field's Bridal Registry. Papà, who had picked me up, told me to enter the house through the front door instead of through the garage. I didn't question him; it never dawned on me that my family would be normal enough to actually invite my friends into our home. But then again, it never dawned on me that we wouldn't realize we weren't normal enough to actually invite people into our home, either.

The entire event was Caterina's idea. I think out of all of us, she probably tried to keep things as close to normal as possible. Or maybe she was the one who just wished them more so into existence. Or maybe she was the one most in denial.

For Christmas, she wanted to go see the department store windows on State Street and spend a day in downtown Chicago shopping—like normal people. In preparation for Easter, she wanted to plant spring flowers, and on the day, she wanted to dress up and go to church—like normal people. She wanted to grow up, get married and have children, a family of her own— like normal people. This surprise party for me was just one more thing she wanted to do that normal people did.

But we weren't normal.

As I walked up to our front door, I did notice for a brief second that our drapes were drawn shut. Usually, they were wide open, and anyone passing by could see the glow of our TV set from inside our living room. I didn't give it much thought. I never put two and two together, and by the time I pushed open our door, it was too late to retreat.

"SURPRISE!"

About a dozen or so of my friends shouted out in unison. They, along with my sister and parents, were in the living room, seated on the floor, our dining room chairs, and our green and gold couches. Even those had been stripped naked of their plastic protectors, something that rarely, if ever, happened. That, maybe, was an even bigger surprise than the actual party surprise.

Caterina took center stage, my own birthday ringmaster, to direct the evening's activities. These included a mandolin serenade by my papà, homemade pizza thanks to Mamma, and the opening of gifts, courtesy of all. One gift in particular stood out: One of my friends had given me the then-popular book *The Joy of Sex*.

Everyone hooted and hollered, and as much as I couldn't wait to read the book, I wasn't so keen on even acknowledging the gift, let alone posing for pictures with it, in front of that entire room. It wasn't so much the book and its topic; rather, it was the fact that I knew I had no real need for it at the moment, and likely wouldn't any time in the near future, either.

My embarrassment only worsened when Papà asked for a translation of the book's title. I pretended not to hear him.

That same year, another surprise came my way, one that was ten years in the making.

When I was eight years old, before heading off to school in the mornings, my siblings and I would turn on the TV to WGN-Channel 9 and start off our day watching *Bozo's Circus*. Uncle Ned, the ringmaster dressed in red tails and a top hat, would open the show by blowing his whistle and announcing, "Bozo's Circus is on the air!" The kids in the audience would cheer and applaud, the marching band would start to play, and Bozo, played by Bob Bell, with his shocking bright red hair, red bulb of a nose, and floppy red shoes, would be introduced as "The world's greatest clown!" to which he'd reply, "Hey, that's me!"

I so wanted to be one of those kids sitting in that studio audience. Tickets were near-impossible to get, but I didn't know that back then. I was determined to see Bozo and his buddies Cooky the Clown and Wizzo the Wizard in person, so I took it upon myself to write into the show, asking for tickets to be sent to me.

Waiting for what seemed like forever, I eventually stopped, and soon afterward I forgot entirely about ever having submitted my request. And then one day, ten whole years later, I got what I had asked for in the mail. So at the age of eighteen, tickets in hand, I, along with my siblings, finally made it to the studio to see *Bozo's Circus* live. It also happened to be one of Bob Bell's final performances as everybody's favorite clown before he retired the following year.

In truth, I hesitated, not quite sure we should go. But Rosario, who had recently turned twenty-one, thought it'd be pretty funny for us to show up, and so we did.

Bob Bell thought it was pretty funny, too. Throughout the taping, he made a point of adlibbing and offering up his own commentary during commercial breaks, saying things that only we could hear. "Blech! If I hear that one more time . . ." Bob as Bozo said while the band played. "I can't stand that song!" He put his fingers down his throat, pretending to gag. We laughed at his distaste for the marching tune and the private jokes he was making and sharing with just us.

Bozo was still Bozo on the outside, but, even at my then-age of eighteen, I understood a little bit of what he must have been feeling. He had pretended for who knows how long to be the jolly clown kids loved—caring for them, making sure they were happy and having a great time during the show. On the inside, however, that wasn't, perhaps, the whole story.

NOW HERE I WAS, TURNING twenty-one years old, far away from home and all of the madness I had grown up with and once again the center of attention in the middle of the unknown.

The build-up to my milestone birthday, the expectations, started to take a toll. It wasn't just the thought of the required bar-hopping celebrations that made me anxious. It had even more to do with where I found myself—with money, my weight, and my love life—versus where I wanted to be.

So to kick off my actual twenty-first birthday, the first surprise to come my way was getting super sick—so ill that I ended up visiting the ISU Health Clinic. I had contracted what felt like some serious flu. Thank God the university's billing department had refused to grant my request to opt-out of medical services on the grounds that I couldn't afford them. Now, as I downed the medication they had prescribed for me, I realized that the mandatory fees were worth it. The potent tonic they had given me clearly stated that consuming liquor alongside it was not allowed. I made no promises, but it was good to know I had an out from any kind of partying if I wanted one.

My family's letters could easily drive me to drink, their birthday card to me notwithstanding.

Papà reminisced about my birth, hoping God would bless me with good health, intelligence, and a love, always, for my family. Oh, and he said tax documents weren't in yet.

Mamma reminded me that she was my mother who gave birth to me.

As if we could forget that fact.

Her doing that isn't normal. Is it?

Cathy, Ross, and Viny all signed off with their wishes.

I couldn't help but laugh, missing them as much as I wished they'd just leave me be. And yet I felt obligated to call and thank them for the birthday greetings.

THE MINUTE I SAID HELLO ON the phone, Papà bit my head off. Something was wrong, and I didn't have it in me to ask what it was. We abruptly ended our chat.

Almost overnight, another letter came with Papà's apology and explanation.

Nello stesso tempo, ti chiedo scusi per il mio arrogante tono di voce quando mi hai telefonato. Cosa vuoi, l'ambiente qui è quasi sempre lo stesso e quindi i miei nervi stanno sempre tesi e, per quanto cerco di frenarmi, delle volte scattano come un automobile a grande velocità e che succede allora? Chi mi capita davanti comprenderà il mio non normale carattere. Comunque, io ti voglio sempre bene e sento davvero la tua mancanza e con me, la sente anche tutta la famiglia.

"At the same time, I ask that you forgive me for my harsh tone when you telephoned. What do you want? The environment here is almost always the same, and so, my nerves are always tense, and as much as I try to control myself, at times, they explode like a speeding car, and then what happens? Whoever happens to be in front of me is subjected to me, out of character. In any event, I always love you and truly miss you, and along with me, the whole family does also."

It wasn't normal for Papà to behave as he had. Crazy corrupts even the strongest among us. I understood, but I didn't have anything left in me just then to ease his angst. Mamma added a few of her own lines at the end of his letter.

Cara Paola - Le polpette quando vieni ti facciamo - Mi auguro che stai bene e non spendere troppo soldi perché l'albero non ne fa assai. Ti abbraccio forte e ti bacio la mamma che sempre ti pensa

Maria Milana

"Dear Paola—The meatballs, when you come, we'll make them. I hope you are well and don't spend too much money, because the tree doesn't make a lot. I hug you tightly and kiss you, your mother who always thinks of you."

Mamma's meatballs were definitely something worth coming home to. She even made me laugh with her money tree quip. Her letter sounded so normal, the opposite of what she usually was. If it wasn't her, then what was causing Papà to act the opposite of *his* normal?

A box arrived. Rosario had sent me a separate surprise: My favorite Mrs. Field's Cookies—chocolate chip, chocolate macadamia, and oatmeal raisin—ten total (I'm sure there had been a full dozen to start with and, knowing my brother, he "taste-tested" two of them). Rosario also shared why the "packing" in the box wasn't the usual Styrofoam peanuts but was a bunch of shredded newspaper *plus* twenty one-dollar bills.

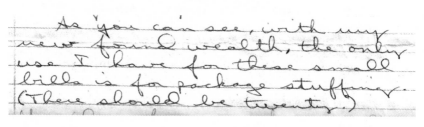

". . . the only use I have for these small bills is for package stuffing . . ."

Funny. As usual. Rosario always found something to laugh about. As appreciative as I was for his gift, I couldn't help but wish he really was rolling in dough, enough to lend me my outstanding tuition. His twenty dollars wasn't going to make much of a dent in the massive debt I had accumulated.

Beth gave me the best birthday surprise: one of her mom's German-chocolate cakes—a dessert I had fallen in love with when staying with her family during Thanksgiving. And Kathy gifted me a giant box of the General Mills Complete Pancake

Mix from her parents' café. Obviously, the girls were in support of my food addictions.

I TURNED TWENTY-ONE ON Wednesday, February 12, 1986. The following Friday was Valentine's Day. Caterina wrote me a separate letter with a plan to help deal with our single statuses.

> a happy subject), How are you set up for
> Feb. 14th? That's Valentine Day, if you're not
> already aware.
>   My Valentine's Day is once again up in the
> air. Bob shows no interest. Tim said he'd call
> hasn't. Gary is obnoxious & Mack likes me,
> but the guy in the white truck might appear
> at any moment to take him away. So Paula,
> I guess our only alternative is to be each others
> valentines, what do you say? It'll be our secret.

At first, I giggled. Then, I was grateful. I was perfectly comfortable with her plan having us be each other's Valentines, and I had mastered the art of keeping secrets, so no issues there. But the more I thought about her proposal, the more I couldn't help but feel like even more of a loser, given the details she'd shared about her own love life. My sister had no less than four guys after her—four living, breathing males who showed potential. Four was four more than I had ever experienced myself.

AS SICK AS I WAS AND AS much as I wasn't supposed to drink while on prescribed medicine, I headed out to the bars in downtown Ames that evening, where I was treated by friends to not just boozy drinks but also a bunch of ice cream. I felt like the queen bee, the toast of the town, and 100 percent, totally free. For those few hours, I made partying my thing, and I could have cared less about anybody other than me.

By the time we returned to our dorm rooms in the wee hours of the morning, I felt as if I had just run a marathon. Not that I would know what that actually felt like, but I had heard about people getting a runner's high, and this, I imagined, was like that.

Until a few hours later, when I was throwing up in the bathroom, wondering what I had done to myself and praying for it to stop.

It wasn't the throbbing headache or the swollen eyes or the parched throat or the upset stomach so much that had me feeling so sick on top of actually being sick. No, it was the feelings of guilt over having let loose and letting go of the people who mattered to me most. After that initial call with Papà being such a grouch, I hadn't bothered to call home again or even take the calls that had come in from home on my birthday. And while the freedom felt fantastic, it also filled me with regret and shame.

You for sure added to your papà's misery.

I imagined I had, and I stewed about it for a few days. I just couldn't bring myself to phone home, because I knew what I would need to do to make things right: pretend.

After my birthday, when I couldn't put it off any longer, I finally phoned, and I told them I hadn't called because I was too sick and had lost my voice. I told them how lonely I was and that I missed them very much. I pretended to feel lost without them, and I cried real tears that nearly convinced even me that I wanted to come home.

Everything about that phone call was a lie. Everything I told them, they believed.

Their letters that followed shamed me even more.

Dear Paula—   2/17/86

Hey, what happened to all of that optimism that you have! Okay, so you are going through a shitty period—we all do (believe me I know, I'm the queen of shitty periods). I understand

But Caterina didn't understand. How could she? Even I didn't understand what was making me feel and behave in this way.

My guilt overcame me when reading the letter from Papà, prompted by my crying to him on the telephone. I could barely get through even his salutation of, "My dearest daughter . . ."

Algonquin Il. 9/18/1986

Mia carissima figlia Paolina,
una sera, prima che tu telefonasi, credimi Paolina,
sentivo il bisogno di parlare con te. In verità io
ti penzo sempre; Domenica per esempio, abbiamo
fatto Pasta fina fina e, nell'ora di pranzo, ho
ditto: Paoletta se la mangerebbe un po di questa
Pasta. cara figlia Paola, io ti vorrei sempre qui vicino
perchè la tua presenza nella famiglia fa sempre
la casa sempre piena e piena di allegria.

Papà wrote that when I called, he was feeling the need to talk with me. In truth, he said, he thought of me always. They had made one of my favorite birthday dishes on Sunday, Pasta Fina Fina. He said he wished I could always be near to him, because, "*La tua presenza nella famiglia fa sembrare la casa sempre piena e piena di allegria*"—"Your presence in the family makes the house seem always full and full of joy."

On the surface, Papà's words were what everyone might want to hear. But the underbelly of Papà's sentiments crystallized what I realized had become my challenge. The pressure of being the upbeat, silver lining, good girl of the family was just too much. Serving as caregiver for so long was siphoning my ability to breathe. I had become just like Bozo. On the outside, I was a performer, the class clown, the family's *consigliere* and source of entertainment. All these years of showing that joyful and take-charge side, and hiding the darker, no-clue parts of me, was proving to be too much. How was I supposed to deal with just me, all of me, when I had everybody else relying on me to help them deal with themselves? And now I had reached a new level of low by faking it. I was actually pretending to cry and care so as to make them feel missed and needed.

That's fucked up.

Or maybe you're just full of yourself.

In ogni modo la telefonata l'ho tanto gradita, ma sono rimasto male sentirti piangere!
Io non voglio affatto che tu piange! Lo so per esperienza di quando ero militare e quando sono stato in Argentina; la lontananza e a volte la solitudine ci fa triste.

"*Io non voglio affatto che tu piange!*"

My papà didn't want me to cry at all. He said he knew what it was like to be homesick, having felt the same when he was in the military and when he went to live in Argentina.

"*La lontananza e a volte la solitudine ci fa triste.*"

But in my case, it wasn't the distance or the solitude that was making me sad. It was the fact that everyone at home expected me to be homesick and feel sad, and I did not. For the most part.

Papà's letter continued.

Poi devi pure pensare che tu non sei mai sola, il pensiero di tuo Papà e sempre vicino a te ed io spero che il sapere questo ti darà coraggio e forza di vincere ogni ostacolo.
Non temere Paola mia! nella scuola qualche volta si male e altre volte bene; se tutto fossi isi nel mondo

*"You are never alone. Your father's thoughts are always
close to you, and I hope that knowing this gives you courage and strength to overcome every obstacle."*

I knew I was never alone. I knew I should be grateful. In so
many ways, it was comforting to have Papà always there for me.
But as much as that was true, it also was true that I found it all to
be suffocating. Call me selfish or thankless or worse—these were
all words I had used myself when considering who I had become.
I couldn't help how I felt, but feeling the way I did, and having
to keep those feelings secret, was driving me to a dark place from
which I feared there would be no return.

I had thought one year of living my own life would be
enough for me to be able to return to the madness of my family.
It wasn't—and now I had only a couple of months left to myself.
The closer my year away came to its close, the farther I distanced
myself from what awaited me at home.

CHAPTER NINE: **CASUALTIES**

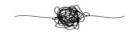

SILENCE: IT HAD BECOME MY choice in communications, or my lack thereof. I hadn't even bothered to call Papà for his birthday in March. I had nothing to say—or at least, nothing good to say. I feared opening my mouth, knowing full well that words wound, especially in the way I had learned to wield them. Before coming to ISU, part of my argument to my papà to get his permission to allow me to go away to school was telling him, "I don't want to end up like you." I hadn't meant it as harshly as it sounded. I meant that I didn't want to break my back every day just to live paycheck to paycheck like he did. But the damage was done.

Feeling the way I felt now, so discouraged at the year coming to an end and knowing that in a few short weeks I'd be heading back to the madness at home, I decided it best to just send a greeting card to my papà. My "Happy Birthday" included the promise that as soon as I did get home, I'd treat him to a birthday dinner at Port Edwards, a seafood restaurant in town that I knew he'd love. It was the best I could do.

I'm sure Papà was hurt. He would have preferred to hear my voice. And it was clear that he had picked up on my attempt to divorce myself from the family. His next letter gently called me out.

Algonquin 3/22/86

Carissima Figlia Paola,
Ti scrivo questa letterina per dimostrarti
che io ti penzo sempre; anche se tu (essendo circon-
data da molte compagne, e anche qualche amica)
credo che non sentirai tanto la lontananza -

"...*io ti penzo sempre; anche se tu (essendo circondata da molte compagne, e anche qualche amica) credo che non sentirai tanto la lontananza.*"

Papà wrote that he thought of me always, even if I, being surrounded by schoolmates and also some friends, didn't feel the same, being far away.

He was right. I didn't miss him or my family, not really. And I didn't relish the thought of returning to them, not at all. My time away and on my own seemed to be doing the exact opposite of what I had hoped. I had gotten a taste of what life was like when I could make myself the priority, be normal (to the extent that I could be), and not have to navigate the madness that had shaped me—and I liked it. I wasn't sure I could go back to the way things were before.

I needed to think. I needed a breather. I wanted to experience just being me. But this little taste of freedom, and the possibility of living my own life had only served to open my eyes to what I feared could never be. Not for me. Like it or not, I was destined to return to madness and to resume my role as caregiver of crazy.

I sighed, forcing myself to read the rest of his letter. Papà continued, explaining to me that on the twenty-first of March, the first day of spring, Viny had attended her last day at the Pioneer Center.

Ti comunico che ieri 21 Marzo (il primo giorno di primavera) è stato l'ultimo giorno di Vincenzina frequentare quella scuola che tu hai suggerito tre mesi fa.

Ti posso assicurare che Vincenzina ha fatto un progresso grande; acquistò qualche amica con la quale si telefona spesso e, già ben due volte, sono uscite assieme (ritirandosi verso le 11 di sera.

What?!

I couldn't believe Papà was pulling her out. It had only been two months.

He assured me that Viny had made great progress. She had even connected with some girlfriends with whom she spoke often on the telephone and had gone out, coming home close to eleven in the evening!

My heart sank. Viny was pulled out much too early. She had just started coming out of her shell. Her first set of friends. Her first taste of freedom and having fun out on the town. *That* was what was normal. *That* was what we all deserved to feel.

Papà knew it, too. I could feel his angst, as he wrote to justify his decision.

In verità l'avrei fatto continuare ancora un paio di mesi; ma come tu sai Vincenzina ha una grande simpatia per quel ragazzo Stefe e poiché Vincenzina non ha affatto esperienza (nella vita...) ho pensato di allontanarla (almeno per un po di tempo) e così calmarla un po di questa primitiva passione.

"In verità l'avrei fatto continuare ..."

He wrote that he would have had her continue, but Viny had become infatuated with a boy named Steve, and Papà wanted to calm her first crush—or as he called it, her "*primitive passione.*" Two more reasons factored into Papà's reasoning for pulling Viny out of the social services. The most important, he wrote, was that Mamma needed companionship to distract her from her thoughts. I scoffed at the notion that Viny was any match for Mamma's mental illness.

L'altra ragione per cui l'ho tolta di quello Istituto (e credo sia importantissimo) la Mamma ha bisogno di compagnia per non pensare tanto

He, too, I'm sure, knew that his plan was faulty at best. But what else could he do? Papà could not stay at home with Mamma, not until he retired. And he couldn't retire until he cleared up a few outstanding bills. But he promised that it wouldn't be much longer before he managed to do so, and that as soon as he could retire, he would stay at home to care for Mamma. In the meantime, he said, to console Viny, who didn't at all want to leave Pioneer Center and her newfound friends, he would pay her ten dollars each week to babysit Mamma.

Vincenzina farà compagnia a Mamma fino che io mi ritiro. Le ho detto che le darò $10 alla settimana per tranquillizzarla, dato che lei non voleva affatto ritirarsi da quello Istituto.

Money. It always seemed to come down to how much we did or didn't have, emphasis on the "didn't" in our case. And when it came to Viny, this would become more costly than any one of us could have known at the time.

Papà shifted back to his unwavering faith in God, referencing that Easter was on the horizon.

Mia bara figlia, domani domenica delle Palme; io e credo tutti andиamo a Messa (di mattina, e verso le ore 13 (1.PM.) batтина e Rosario, vogliono che andиamo al Ristorante P. Edward.

Sono sicuro che la spesa toccherà pagarla il (Babbo). e così festeggeremo il compleanno. Mi Piacerebbe che ci fossi anche tu; ma io aspetto il tuo ritorno per godere di quel Pranzo che mi hai promesso nella cartolina. Ti Bacio affettuosamente, tuo Padre

— Buona Pasqua — Antonino Milacca

THE FAMILY PLANNED TO GO to mass on Palm Sunday and, of course, Easter Sunday, with dinner following at Port Edwards. Papà assumed he would have to foot the bill; joking, he called himself "*Babbo,*" which in Italian translates both to "father" and "idiot." I laughed.

He closed by saying that he awaited my return, since I had promised to treat him to a meal at Port Edwards, and that he would enjoy it being just us.

With every line I read, my heart sank further.

Mamma's note followed. She, too, wished me a happy Easter. Her penmanship, always a dead giveaway as to whether or not she was on her meds, proved to me that she was on.

Cara Paola — se non ci Vediamo per Pasqua ti auguro di passarla bene anche se non siamo assieme cerca di essere contenta che la Pasqua si può fare pure dopo ti bacio la mamma

"*. . . se non ci vediamo per Pasqua ti auguro di passarla bene anche se non siamo assieme cerca di essere contenta che la Pasqua si può fare pure dopo . . .*"

She encouraged me to be happy, even if we wouldn't be together for Easter.

I let out a sigh. How could I be honest about the fact that I was happy, in great part, *because* we would *not* be together for Easter?

You really need to go to confession.

Confession? Do I need to explain again how my last time went?

That was then. This is now.

Palm Sunday was the coming weekend, and then Easter followed. I loved Easter and what it stood for: rebirth, renewal, resurrection. Maybe it was time to give God another shot.

A CATHOLIC CHURCH NAMED FOR a saint I had never heard of was the closest to campus. St. Thomas Aquinas was about a half-mile from my dorm. It would take a normal person ten minutes or so to walk there—but my less-than-speedy pace was nowhere near normal, so I headed out on Palm Sunday just after sunrise to make sure I made it on time, and have almost an hour to check the place out before mass actually got started. That's what I really wanted to do: roam around and investigate without anybody asking questions.

From the outside, St. Thomas Aquinas didn't look much like a church. It reminded me more of a grade school, with its pinkish brick and cottage-like windows. I wondered if they held classes or something on the second floor. As I looked up, I noticed what I guessed was supposed to be its steeple, though no stretch of the imagination could turn it into one. The front entrance rose to a triangular peak and up on the very tip teetered the tiniest metal cross.

I climbed the steps and pulled open one of the giant glass entrance doors. Inside, a couple of long tables draped in white cloth had been set up. Row after row of fresh green palm leaves were neatly laid out for inspection and, I assumed, selection by parishioners to take home following the service. My papà was a master at weaving our palms into patterns and different shapes. Every Palm Sunday, I'd watch him transform fat green reeds into braided leaves and ribbons that looked like a cross and—my favorite—a pine cone–looking basket that he'd give to me to put over the corner of the mirror in my room. He'd tried to teach me the art of palm weaving, but I'd never quite managed to match his level of expertise.

"*A la terza si libbira,*" Papà would say—"third time's the charm"—another of his favorite Sicilian proverbs that he used to fit any occasion. He practically raised us on those proverbs. Most of the time, he'd have to explain each word. More than just a dialect, Sicilian seemed to be its own language. Though Italian was my native tongue, I couldn't understand Sicilian. But the sound of those proverbs were so musical and, often, unforgettable. My all-time favorite was "*Dimmi con chi vai e ti dirò chi sei.*" Translation? "Tell me who you go with and I'll tell you who you are."

Who was I? With whom did I run? In the quiet of that moment, I realized I hadn't a clue. I took care of others. I was the reluctant caregiver. And now I was becoming a resentful one.

I chose three of the palms from the table, just in case I really did need three tries to get one right. I would try my hand at palm weaving, keep the best of the three, and give the other two to Beth and Kathy.

Carrying my palms like a baby cradled in my arms, I entered the main part of the church. No one was inside yet. At the very front was what I guessed was the sanctuary, though it seemed to be missing the typical white marble altar. Did churches no longer use them? Where was the pulpit?

After taking just a few steps down the center aisle, I genuflected beside the very last row and slid into the pew to sit. Quietly, I set down my palms to my right and reached down to pull out the kneeler. I hated when we had to kneel during mass. The pads didn't really help with comfort. But since it was Palm Sunday, out of respect for God, and as penance for not having visited Him on my own for a private chat in—wow—maybe seven or eight years, I thought I would try.

I folded my hands in prayer and leaned forward to kneel—and immediately regretted the decision to do so. The moment my knees made contact with the hard wood, I thought back to when the nuns in grammar school made me kneel on pencils as punishment. What I had done to deserve that, I couldn't even remember.

There's no way God's only going to listen on the condition you kneel in pain.

I agreed. If God really was all-loving, would it matter to Him whether or not I knelt? I pushed back and chose to take my chances seated.

In the nothingness, my own breathing sounded so loud. Only the cavernous echo of the occasional tiny pings and creaks pierced the silence.

"Are you there, God? It's me, Margaret." Why Judy Blume's book came to mind, I wasn't sure. And I sure did hope God knew it was me, Paula—or Paolina, if we were going to be formal with reintroductions.

You're being really stupid.

I laughed, because I was.

A jolt of music suddenly started to play, startling me. I looked around, figuring somebody must be doing sound checks in preparation for the service. No one was around that I could see. I listened to the song playing. It was one I had not heard before. I couldn't quite understand its words: It sounded as if they were saying "Kyrie Lay-son" and something about the road less traveled? Or no, the road I *must* travel.

Moments later, the people fiddling with the music started talking. I still couldn't see them, but their chatter was making it difficult to hear the lyrics. They stopped speaking, and then they started the song again.

Birds or some sort of chirping, louder and louder, and then those words: Kyrie Lay-son, Kyrie Lay ... or E-lay-son? Something about being between your soul. I tried to keep up with the lyrics, but found myself struggling. I could catch some words here and there: "Will you follow," "darkness of the night," "young and old," "chosen road," and "what I wished that I could be . . ."

Before I even realized what was happening, tears had flooded my eyes.

The chorus boomed, repeating "Kyrie Eleison" over and over; it reverberated off the church's walls and windows. I could feel the tingle of vibrations within me.

Why are you crying?

I had no idea. And now people had started crowding inside: families, couples, groups of friends. Everyone had someone. Everyone except me.

I quickly raised my hand to wipe away the tears spilling down my cheeks.

How embarrassing.

You're a mess.

I grabbed my palm leaves and, before anyone could see me and my blubbering self, exited the pew, clumsily genuflected, apologized to God for not sticking it out, and left the building.

Kyrie Eleison: I kept repeating the words in my head, not wanting to forget them so I could find the song and research their meaning once I got back to my dorm. I kept my gaze directed downward, focusing on my two feet and the pavement, trying to avoid anyone seeing the tears that I just couldn't seem to stop from flowing.

IN THE SILENCE OF MY OWN dorm room, I sat on my bed, tears still welling up in my eyes. I had no idea what those words meant or why that song or sitting in that church had hit me the way they had. All alone, I allowed myself to feel whatever it was I was feeling. And I picked up my palms and started weaving.

Later, I can't recall when, I would learn that those three words were Greek and translated to "Lord, have mercy." I also would become known on the dorm floor for the creations I had made out of those Palm Sunday reeds. It took me three tries on the same design, but the last pine cone basket weave was nearly perfect. Only Papà and God and I would know its flaws.

THE FINAL WEEKS OF THAT spring semester seemed like just days, the very opposite of what Papà had said he felt shortly after dropping me off at school the previous August. Thoughts of heading back home permanently weighed on my mind. When Lee surprised our class by asking us to write her an impromptu update of our final projects and our overall thoughts about her non-fiction creative writing class, what spilled out of me and onto the page made me hesitate over whether I should actually turn it in to her.

> I would never want anyone to know how much you can hate someone. But, I feel the need to explain to people that you can wish a schizophrenic parent dead when they are at their worst and then love them so much when they're having a good day — that sometimes you think you're going crazy. I don't know, does any of this make sense. Maybe I am going crazy.

Clearly, I had lost my mind. Telling Lee I wanted to write about how you could love someone and at the same time wish them dead...? What was I doing? Unfortunately, there was no time for a rewrite, so hand it in I did.

I also wrote my update on our "Glimpses" assignment. I'd told her that I had decided to do the piece on the "Dieter's World." I'd written, "I haven't had much success in dieting, but that doesn't mean I don't have the experience. I've probably followed every diet there is. Now if only I could just stick to it longer than three days."

Maybe your genes aren't just crazy but fat, too.

I nodded in agreement.

The final paper—"Glimpses of a Dieter's World"—included a "Dieter's Vocabulary" with amusing definitions of words known to those of us carrying around extra baggage. I wrote down "Diet:

The ultimate in self-denial. Refusing entrance through the mouth to one's favorite foods. Root word—DIE." Snippets of "Dieter's Dreams" and "Dieter's Nightmares" called out visions of double chocolate brownies juxtaposed against steamed carrots. "Dieter's Exercises" offered up ridiculous explanations of movements such as "Jaw Flexes: Slowly and with care open mouth as wide as possible, hold four seconds, close mouth quickly and relax. Benefit: Eases jaw tension when trying to pack more food into mouth than mouth was made to hold." I concluded with a section called "Lies Dieters Tell Themselves." I had used several of these throughout my own dieting career: "Just one more," and "I was good all day, so I can have this," and "Please, God, just let me wake up tomorrow thin."

Please, God, don't let me be like Mamma.

A letter from Mamma came in the mail. I had thought to use it in the piece I had promised to Lee as part of what I intended to write as one of my final projects.

Mamma tried to explain her own loss of self and utter sense of failure in her letter. She wrote of how happy she had been, once upon a time, with her own business as a seamstress and dressmaker. She talked about little party dresses she had been making for twin toddlers, and the joy she'd felt sewing tiny bells into the layers of poufy netting and tulle that made up their tea-length skirts. Mamma's client list kept growing, she wrote, but her illness had as well—and it had ultimately put a stop to her even being able to make good on promised delivery dates. Eventually, she'd no longer felt good enough to do anything.

"Ecco, che aggravandomi."

"How exasperating for me," she wrote.

I imagined Mamma sitting down to write her letter, her truth, her pain, her sorrow. All of her dreams, too, had been halted just as they were getting started. Her frustration loomed forth from the page, every stroke of her pen a cry that asked, why? Who was orchestrating her demise? To whom should she point her finger for ruining her life and that of her family? Who was responsible for this thing she was so powerless to control?

Mamma's letter forced me to realize that she, too, was a victim of her disease. She wasn't at fault, any more than any one of us was. Still, we all needed someone to blame. Mamma blamed the doctors, Papà, and us. For me, Mamma was the easiest target.

I could not bring myself to write about Mamma as part of Lee's final assignment. Instead, I wrote about Papà. I called his piece "A Special Someone's Murphy's Law Day" and shared the story of what happened when I went home for Christmas. I focused on a different kind of madness—my papà's brush with the law due to his driving the wrong way on a one-way street, after waking up late and racing to get to work—and I chose to spin it to a magical conclusion.

Having turned my work in to both Lee and Dr. Mack, and having taken my final exams, I spent my remaining days on campus saying my good-byes to Janet and Marie and Charlie the cadaver. I also visited my hawk with no name that still fought to free herself from her cage, not knowing enough about her own condition to realize that doing so might be the death of her in the end. I groomed Charlie the horse for the last time, and didn't even fight him when he insisted on eating my hair.

When I returned to my dorm room, more letters had come for me.

Io penzo che qualche tasca del buon pantalone sarà bucata e i soldi li perde . . . . è vero?

"Some pockets of your trousers I think have holes in them and you're losing your money . . . is that true?" Papà joked.

I laughed, thinking, *If only that was the problem.* Truth was, my problem was much bigger. I wouldn't be getting my grades, because I still owed Iowa State a couple thousand dollars for tuition and fees. I had called Rosario and told him this, and he, according to Papà's letter, had passed on the news of my lack of funds. Papà wrote that Rosario would be sending me some money—and he did, but it was pretty much pocket change. I hadn't let on even to my brother exactly how much money I needed.

You still have a few days.

Still having a few days didn't matter when I had no idea how to get that kind of cash in hand. I would have no choice but to visit the people in the ISU Financial Aid offices.

I pretended all was well with Beth and Kathy, celebrating our farewells by charging to my credit card even more merriment while out in the town's bars. Then I did it all again the following night with Shelly. I charged last-minute, ISU-branded stuff I didn't need, and after selling back my textbooks, I blew the money on late-night fast-food orders at Hardee's: charbroiled burgers and fries for my friends, on me!

Big city, big spender: That was what I wanted to be known for. That was the new image I was creating for myself. That was part of my being normal. Not the fat girl. Not the poor chick. And definitely not the one with insanity genes.

THE LAST DAY OF MY WRITING class included a one-on-one meeting with Lee. I'm not sure she had them with everybody, but she did with me.

When I walked into her tiny office, she wasn't sitting on top of her desk as she did during class; rather, she sat in her chair like a grownup. Still, underneath that mop of silvery hair, I could see the mischievous grin of her twelve-year-old inner child. I chuckled a bit—not just at the smile but at the piles of papers, overstuffed manila folders, and books, so many books, that surrounded her.

Lee looked at me looking at her mess, then dramatically threw her hands up in the air and waved me in: "'If a cluttered desk is a sign of a cluttered mind, of what, then, is an empty desk a sign?'" she quoted from memory. "If it's good enough for Einstein, it's good enough for me!"

I nodded, laughing. I loved everything about her.

"Sit, sit," she said as she rose from her chair and came around the front of her desk to sit on its edge, right in front of me.

After easing myself into one very skinny, vinyl, bucket-like chair and plopping my backpack onto its empty twin beside me, I looked up at Lee. Her reassuring smile put me at ease and made me feel as if this was where I belonged.

She handed me my two final papers, her comments scribbled onto each. She had showered me with words of praise and said that I should try to sell them to publications. My heart raced as I read her words of encouragement, and upon realizing she had given me an A not just for both papers but for the class overall.

> —I think what you should write is a piece about this marvelous man — not confined to just one day — I think you should push the editorial quality — I think you should try to sell it —
>
> A Special Someone's Murphy's Law Day.

We chatted more about the book she had written. I so wanted to ask Lee if she was really twelve-year-old Abby, but I didn't. She shared that it hadn't been easy for her and her writing partner to get the book written, let alone published. And then she said words I never imagined I would hear: "Paolina, I don't say this to too many of my students, but you were born to write. And I hope it's what you choose to do with your life."

I can't recall much else from that meeting. What I do remember is the feeling I had of finally having some direction, a goal, a purpose. I wasn't just about money, dieting, and mental illness. I was a writer. Lee thought I was good enough for someone to pay me to write. She saw me not as just "normal" but as somebody *special*. Her encouragement was what I needed to be able to survive going home for good.

ON THE LAST DAY PAYMENT could be made for outstanding monies owed to the school so that they would release grades and transcripts, I headed out to meet with ISU's financial counselors. On my way, I stopped by my mailbox and found three more letters.

Dear "Poor" Paula: Monday

My husband put a request for
settlement of your case before we
left so he should be hearing soon.
Will send your check for a "million"
as soon as we get it.

We MISS you

Hope all will be well
at your Home — sorry
about every thing Lost & Stuff
Idelle (mrs Stone)

The first one I opened was from Mrs. Stone who advised me that her attorney husband had put in the request for settlement on my food poisoning case and said that they would send my "check for a million" soon.

We wish!

I agreed.

And then I saw the second letter. Its return address was from the law offices of her husband. I tore the envelope open. While it wasn't a check for a million dollars, it *was* a check for a few thousand dollars—enough for *all* of my outstanding university tuition and fees, plus a few dollars more.

I stuttered in my step, nearly tripping. My school debt had just evaporated. Realization swept over me as I kissed that check and apologized to fate. The very thing I had cursed back in August—getting food poisoning—was the very reason I now had in my hands the money I needed to pay for school.

My entire body relaxed. The noose around my neck loosened. Gravity no longer seemed to have hold of me. Looking up at the heavens, I felt as if I could float right up to the sky and ride one of its billowy clouds to anywhere. "Thank you!" I spoke the words out loud. "To you who helped orchestrate this little twist, sincerest thanks!"

Moments later, I was on my way, practically skipping down the path, to the ISU Treasurer's Office to finally have "Paid in Full" stamped on my university bill.

As I happily waited in line, I opened the third letter.

May 5, 1986

Dear Paula,

You don't know me, but I know you
pretty well. You are the pretty young girl
that lived across the street from my Dad.
You are the girl he was worrying about if
you didn't have a date Saturday night. (He
worried about my sisters the same way)
You are the young lady that always brought
a smile to Dad's face and had something
nice to say all the time. Paula, your kindness and caring gave Dad much pleasure.
I know because Dad told me about you and
asked me to write explaining why he had
not been able to answer your last letter.

Thank you & God bless you

Ted Austin Jr.

My smile dissolved as I digested the words. Ted Austin, Jr. had written me a letter. It took me a minute to put two and two together, to even make the connection that Ted was Mr. Austin's son, despite them having the very same name. I sucked in my breath when my brain finally kicked in.

"Dad told me about you and asked me to write why he had not been able to answer your earlier letter."

Ted was trying to explain, and while he clearly couldn't bring himself to even write the words, "My dad is dead," I knew that was what he needed to share.

My honorary grandpa, Mr. Austin, had died.

I swallowed back the lump in my throat that had formed. My momentary feelings of lightness returned to their previous weighty state. I had meant to visit Mr. A when I went home for Christmas, but I hadn't. It had never dawned on me that it might be my last chance to see him and to talk to him.

Had he died alone? Had he been surrounded by Mrs. Austin and all their children? Had he known how much he had meant to me for so many years, first living across the street and then writing me his letters this last year? Was he the angel who'd made it possible for me to get the money I needed before my time ran out?

I had no answers. Looking up at the ceiling lights, hoping to stop the spill of tears, I thanked Mr. Austin for what he had been to me and made a promise to try and do as he said: "Always stay nasty."

Part Two:
The End of The Beginning

*"If you do not change direction, you may
end up where you are heading."*
—LAO TZU

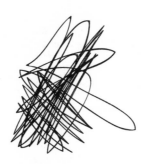

CHAPTER TEN: **CONFUSION**

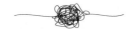

May 1986

.

I WAS BACK AT HOME.

Only it didn't feel like home. It wasn't *my* home.

When I had left for college, we'd lived in a split-level four-bedroom house in Skokie, a suburb just outside of Chicago. Now, not even 365 days later, I was expected to call this three-bedroom, barn-like house in Algonquin, Illinois, a forty-mile drive northwest of the city home—and I couldn't yet bring myself to do that. About the only thing Skokie and Algonquin had in common was their Native American tribal names. And, of course, my crazy family.

Who you callin' crazy?

Good point. I wasn't yet sure how far, if far at all, I had fallen from the family tree. All I was sure of was that everyone else had had months to make this place their home. I had just gotten there. So adjusting to my new environment would take some time.

That was completely normal.

I already had known about Algonquin for a while. It was where Port Edwards tempted seafood lovers and sailors to its doors (I being the former but definitely not the latter). With its rotted-looking wooden-planked exterior, the eatery seemed to float on the edge of the Fox River. With no other dining options around, it reigned over the waterfront, the sailboats, the summer cottages, the tiny docks, and the lucky people for whom this was normal.

Before, the countryside look and feel of Algonquin would have been a little bit of heaven, a place I would have wanted to escape to. But now, it was the place that the very people and things from which I wanted to escape resided.

Algonquin had a lot to offer, including horses and cows that shared the neighborhood and, just behind our new home, a paved trail that stretched from one end of our town to a place called Crystal Lake that sounded very inviting. I envisioned a sparkling jewel sitting at the end of the road, sort of like the Wizard of Oz's Emerald City, if you just followed that yellow-brick road. It sounded so pretty, in fact, that I committed myself to hopping on my bicycle, pedaling the six miles or so, and visiting the spot—one day, when I had skinnied down to the munchkin-size proportions I would need to possess in order to take such a trip.

Homes sat on bigger lots here, much bigger than those closer to the city. My papà rejoiced at our giant backyard and was already plowing and planting the earth to give birth to what would become his envy-worthy vegetable garden. Now sixty-nine and semi-retired, Papà spent the bulk of his days digging in the dirt and encouraging his seedlings to grow. Tomatoes, basil, broccoli, peppers, eggplants, zucchini—his green thumb could make anything grow. And here, he had so much more room with which to use it.

He had even planted a white wine grape called the Muscat of Alexandria. He had gotten the seeds through the mail, a gift from his childhood friend back in Sicily. His "ancient vine" had no business growing in the harsh climate of Midwestern winters, but Papà had faith that with the right amount of care, he would one day soon be able to harvest his own juicy grapes and turn them into the sweet wine of his homeland.

When I came home, the seedlings had barely begun to take root and rise up out of the ground, with just a few green tendrils coiling their way around the silver chain link fence that rimmed our property. Papà would gently caress the tiny leaves that struggled to climb and say, *"Guarda, Paolamia, che biscotti potrebbe fare la mamma con questo vino dolce?"*

I loved when Papà called me "his Paola" and shared his dreams of what might be. Papà asking about the kinds of cookies Mamma might bake from his sweet wine, despite the fact that it would take a couple of years for even the first grapes to emerge, was typical of his hopeful heart. Already, he envisioned us savoring the fruits of his harvest well before anybody else even believed they'd take root.

He also believed in a future that included Mamma returning to her love of creating, whether cooking or sewing. I had abandoned such hopes. It was too painful to wish for what seemed likely to never be.

Mamma spent the majority of her days inside, out of the sunlight and under the covers. She would be turning sixty in July of that year, yet her slow-moving body and her drug-dimmed spirit seemed so much older. Her mental illness continued to rob her of any kind of joy or peace. We had moved into this new home because she had begged for a fresh start, away from the hallucinations and voices she feared. Unfortunately, her paranoid schizophrenic mind had come along for the ride, as it always did, with all of its baggage still threatening to do harm and to put Mamma (if not the rest of us) underground, planted in an early grave.

I still feared those voices.

You have voices, too, ya know?

"They're not the same," I argued back.

How do you know?

I ignored the constant question—not only because I didn't know the answer, but because I had no desire to entertain any possibilities. I tried my best to act as if the voices in my head were more normal than not. They had to be. And I prayed every single night to a God I wasn't sure was even listening that time would speed up.

"Please don't make me like Mamma," I begged.

I asked for Him to end my twenties sooner rather than later and turn me over to a new decade—that magical age of thirty—when

I would know for sure that the insanity genes had kindly passed me by. The doctors had told us that schizophrenia usually hit in one's twenties. They said that Mamma's onset of the disorder in her late forties was rare and that she had quite possibly had symptoms earlier but managed to hide them from others. Or, they surmised, perhaps some traumatic event—like the unexpected death of Mamma's brother, Uncle Joe—had incited the psychosis.

In my opinion, however, those doctors—the same ones who, in 1981, had first performed brain surgery on Mamma, thinking her symptoms were physical and not mental—were clueless and useless. So when these same medical professionals finally diagnosed Mamma with paranoid schizophrenia and then stated that schizophrenia was *not* hereditary, I didn't believe them.

Before Mamma got sick, she'd told fantastical stories of her aunts and older siblings back in Sicily being visited by visions or spirits. She'd also shared how her father had been beaten by someone or something not visible to anyone else as punishment for refusing his eldest daughter Lucia's wishes to become a nun. Mamma was deeply religious, and often made the sign of the cross for no reason I could see. At the same time, she was superstitious—believed in white magic and the evil eye. She feared it all, and I had come to realize that she had good reason to. It was clear: Our family history was riddled with hearing and seeing things that didn't really exist. And the odds were not in our favor that one of us wouldn't be next in line to inherit the insanity genes.

I was determined that it wasn't going to be me, however—not if I could help it. And I knew what I had to do: stay vigilant and mindful and keep my distance from Mamma and her madness.

As for my siblings, the older two were in and out, working and living their own lives as best they could. For them, this new home was little more than a place to crash. Rosario, who was now twenty-four, inhabited the entire downstairs recreation room. He enjoyed his own bathroom and shower and slept on a king-size waterbed he had set up in the corner. He hung his clothes on a Z-rod on wheels and a couple of plywood shelves served as his dresser drawers. Caterina, now twenty-five, set up her own space in the tiniest of the home's three bedrooms. In that eleven-foot by eight-foot space, she managed to arrange furniture in a way that, to me, made it look more like a little apartment than just a bedroom. Her day bed, with its antique-looking brass frame, served as a little loveseat when she wasn't sleeping in it. I envied the bed and her elder status, meaning she automatically got her own bedroom.

I, on the other hand, as the middle daughter, found myself with no other choice but to share an eleven-foot by nine-foot bedroom with Viny. Rather than pretty day beds, Viny and I slept in child-size bunk beds; it was the only way for two grown bodies to occupy such a tiny space and still have room to move. Bunking had been a fun experience and just fine while living in ISU's dorms. Coming home for Christmas and spending a couple of weeks not sleeping in a real bed also had been tolerable. But now, having to officially sleep in the bottom bunk at the age of twenty-one with my nineteen-year-old sister up above—and knowing that this would be the case for as long as I lived at home—proved less than ideal. The lack of privacy alone was depressing. And the fact that I still hadn't found my stuff from the old house, despite having asked repeatedly what might have happened to it during the move, only furthered my feelings that this house wasn't my home and that I didn't belong.

That planted the seed in my brain to get out and find a place of my own as soon as I could afford to.

The challenge, as always, was money. I still had more than $8,000 in credit card debt to pay off from my time at school. For what, exactly, I wasn't even sure. All I knew was that I didn't have the finances to continue with college, at least not for right now. My only choice was to take a year off, find a job, and work until I had enough in my bank account to finish my education.

FORTUNATELY FOR ME, I SOON landed a full-time position at a company that manufactured and sold photocopiers. What, exactly, a "credit correspondent" was supposed to do I hadn't a clue—but the people in charge decided I could do it, so I accepted the position.

I had been given my own desk and calculator, but what I immediately fell in love with was the IBM Selectric Typewriter. At about two feet wide, it took up nearly the entire desktop. It also weighed almost forty pounds, so trying to move it around wasn't going to happen easily. But that didn't matter. I wanted it front and center. The keys almost shimmered, as if they had never been touched. I typed eighty-five words per minute, and I couldn't wait to let my fingers fly each day.

I kept to myself there, trying to do the job I was hired to do. Papà would come and have lunch with me from time to time. He'd pack some healthy, Weight Watchers–compliant dish, and we would sit at one of the picnic tables on the grounds of the offices and gobble it up.

"*Se potessi perdere dieci chili, i ragazzi ti starebbero intorno!*"

All I had to do, according to Papà, was lose ten kilos, about twenty-five pounds, and the boys would surround me.

"*Che pensi?*" he asked.

He always wanted to know what I was thinking. More often than not, I didn't want him to know what was really going on in my head. What could I say to his repeated reminder that I was not skinny enough to attract boys? Why would I even share with him that I had a major crush on my coworker? How could I tell him that it was unfair that we didn't have enough money for me to finish school? Who would he think me to be if I told him I was sick of being the caregiver kid—*la piccola Mamma*—and even more sick of Mamma and all her madness? When would I be able to tell him that I wished I was any place but where I found myself to be?

Seriously? You can't add to his burden.

I settled on answering him with the one word I often used when asked "what's wrong?" or "what are you thinking?"

"*Niente, Papà.*"

Nothing to see here.

SHARING A ROOM WITH VINY meant I didn't have my own room to escape to, unless she wasn't around. So every Saturday and Sunday, I found myself only too happy to wake up early and volunteer to drive her to her job at Bishop's Buffet near Spring Hill Mall in West Dundee. The McHenry County Services empowerment classes she'd stopped taking before she'd really even started had motivated her enough to apply, all on her own, to jobs at the local restaurants. This one had hired her first as waitstaff, but after they'd realized she couldn't get the diners' food orders right and dropped more dirty dishes than she cleaned, they'd moved her into the only position she *was* able to handle: silverware roller. Her one mission was as the title implied: take one fork, one spoon, and one knife, make sure they were clean, and tightly roll them up into burgundy-colored cloth napkins. Hour after hour, that was all she did.

You'd blow your brains out doing that.

Viny hated the job. I rejoiced that she *had* a job. At least now she had a little bit of money that was all her own, had a chance at making friends, and wasn't stuck inside the house all by herself with Mamma.

"How much have you saved so far, Vince?" I asked one day when dropping her off in front of the restaurant's entrance.

"Not enough," she replied in a frustrated tone.

"How about we take a vacation somewhere once you have enough money? I'll even match you dollar for dollar."

"Yeah, yeah." Sweat was already beaded on her face as she pushed open her passenger-side door. Her uniform—polyester black pants and a burgundy polo and apron—had me sweating just looking at it.

As she exited my car, I cheerily reminded her, "Another day, another dollar."

Viny turned and, just before slamming the car door shut, smirked at me and said, "Yeah, but for me it's, 'Another day, another 50 cents.'"

I watched as she moseyed on in, feeling helpless. What could I possibly do to help her?

She's not your kid.
She ain't your problem.

WHILE THE WAY I HAD COME, Route 31, was windy and more scenic, Route 25 was faster and more direct. Hunger made speed my priority, so for the ride home, I chose the latter. There was a point along that road, however, where I couldn't help but slow down: the place where a Dominick's Finer Foods grocery store sat on one side of the street and the Dundee Township Cemetery sat on the other. No matter what else was going on in my head, I couldn't help but hear the words Papà always said whenever he was in the car with me and we came to that point: *"Quando muoio, mi potete mettere lì, così potete salutarmi ogni volta che fate la spesa."*

I would always laugh it off. But his request to be buried in that cemetery so that we could say hello to him every time we went grocery shopping wasn't all that funny. I never wanted to think of the day when he would no longer be at my side. We were more than just a father and his daughter; he was my lifeline to living and laughing and loving, no matter the madness that surrounded us.

AS I ROLLED INTO OUR DRIVEWAY, I could see my papà out in the back working in his vegetable garden. Actually, I could only see his backside in those blue-and-black-checked shorts he loved and always wore. His butt pointed straight up in the air as he hunched over—pulling, I assumed, stubborn weeds out from in between his precious plants.

After putting my car in park and turning off the engine, I hopped out, entered the yard through the little gate, and crossed in front of the shed, making my way over to where he stood.

The fragrant smells of the basil he had planted scented the summer breeze. The sun beat down brightly, causing me to put one hand over my eyes and squint. Papà straightened up, turned toward me, and smiled, his entire face beaming just as bright.

With a gardening trowel in one hand and a fistful of weeds in the other, he raised both arms and gestured to the growing fruits of his labor. He pointed out plants to me, telling me about each one's destiny: tomato plants sprouting red balls of what would become homemade *Bolognese*; bulbous purple eggplants and green peppers that would marry into a spicy *caponata*; and Sicilian zucchini, or *cucuzza*, that dangled from a wooden fence and clothesline contraption Papà had constructed to help the squash grow long enough to resemble a saxophone, would be used in one of my favorite pastas that Mamma made.

Papà exhaled joyously. "*Mi fa cantare il cuore!*"

His vegetable garden made his heart sing.

It made me happy that he was so happy.

"Hey, Mushroom Man . . ."

The gruff voice startled us both.

Papà looked past me as I turned to follow his gaze. "Rich! You come early," he said, and moved quickly in his black socks and white tennis shoes to greet the man he affectionately called "my buddy."

"Agh, this stupid leg wouldn't let me sleep." Rich rapped his callused knuckles a few times on his plastic prosthetic. "I figured 'Tony's probably already in his garden,' so I just got in the car and I'm here."

"Two minoots and we go," Papà said.

The pair shared a laugh and leisurely made their way back to the garden, back to where I still stood. "Rich, this is my Paolina."

"Hey!" the six-foot giant boomed as he awkwardly shook my hand. "Your pop talks about you all the time. You look just like him."

I raised my eyebrows at his remark. "Papà talks about you, too."

I had heard it so many times before: spitting image of Papà—or, as Papà would say, reincarnation of his mother, my grandmother, *la nonna*. As always, I wondered what, exactly, was meant by this comparison. After all, I was far from being bald or toothless like Papà, and while I weighed more than a couple hundred pounds, *la nonna* had weighed in at nearly 500 pounds. Neither lookalike option seemed like something to celebrate.

"Are you guys going mushroom hunting again?" I asked.

"Too early," said Papà. "*Funghi* come in fall." He folded his barrel-like frame and began to gather a few green peppers, egg-plant, and tomatoes. "*Paolamia, vai prendere un sacchetto per Papà.* I give some vege-TAbles to Rich."

I nodded and turned to retrieve a bag for Papà.

"No, Tony." Rich offered in weak protest. "It's too much."

"S-s-s-st!" Papà hissed as he continued his collection. "*Paola,* go. *Sono nel capannone.*"

Without further discussion, I jogged over to the end of the yard just inside the gate, toward the shed. Its door was open. I realized I had never actually checked out the inside before. Entering the storage unit, I saw all sorts of tools hanging on its inside walls, the paper sacks Papà had wanted me to bring to him, our lawn mower, and then, stacked one on top of the other, three somewhat smashed boxes, each with my name written on the sides in thick black lettering.

I pulled open the top of one of the boxes. Inside, I could see my missing things, including my vinyl records, carelessly tossed within. I pulled one out: Billy Ocean's *Loverboy*. It was totally warped, destroyed. From what I could see, all my records had suffered the same fate.

"*Paola*!"

Hearing Papà cry out for me, I tossed the ruined record back into the box, wondering what else I would find in the other two. I grabbed a paper sack and hustled back to Papà and Rich.

"*Ecco,* Papà." I so wanted to rage at him, but I couldn't do it just then. How could he have allowed all of my stuff to just be tossed aside, as if it didn't matter? As if *I* didn't matter enough to care for what mattered to me while I was at school?

I held open the sack as my father carefully filled it with some of his garden's finest. After emptying his arms, he took the bulg-ing package from me and handed it to Rich.

"You give to your wife, eh?" Papà smiled and winked at Rich, who struggled to keep hold of the heavy bag while balancing on his one good leg. Papà had told me once that Rich was lucky he still had a wife, for when the fifty-five-year-old lost his leg in a boating accident, he'd also lost his job and most of his friends, and his wife had threatened to leave. Papà said that Rich had lost his spirit that day. What he didn't say was that he considered it his mission to help him get it back. Not a surprise. And judging by the smile on Rich's face, Papà was on track to succeed.

And you're pissed off about some replaceable records?

Rich settled the bag in one arm and shifted his weight for better balance. "We'll make some minestrone, Tony, the 'PO-lock' way, and you come eat at my house."

Papà laughed. "Good deal." He picked up the water hose that snaked at his feet and sprayed the earth from his hands, then shot a spray at me. It only furthered my silent stewing. After clapping his hands twice to dry them, he said to Rich, "Okay, now we go. Paola, tell Mamma I come back."

I couldn't help but soften as I watched Papà and Rich heading out on their adventure like a couple of teenage boys on their way to beat the block's record at the video arcade. *Of course, you'll be back*, I thought. *You always come back.*

"And if Mamma wants to know where you went?" I asked.

Without turning to answer, Papà shouted with a giggle, "Tell she we go to flea *marketta*."

"The flea market?" I murmured to myself as I leisurely followed the pair out of the yard and toward the driveway. I stopped to lean against the outside of the shed, shrugged, and smiled, watching the duo slide themselves into Rich's monster of a car, then waved them off until they drove out of sight.

Standing in the quiet of the moment, I shut my eyes and turned my face upward to feel the sun's rays. At least Papà seemed happy.

"Antonino?"

I heard Mamma's weak voice calling out for Papà. Slowly, I opened my eyes. It was still so early, not even 8:00 a.m. Why was Mamma up already?

"Antonino . . ." my mother's trembling voice repeated. "*Dové sei?*"

Letting out a sigh, I pushed off from the shed and began to make my way up the front steps and into our house to answer Mamma's call. My stuff, strewn in those boxes, had waited months to be discovered; what harm would a few more hours or days do? Everything was ruined anyway.

As I climbed the stairs up to the living room, I responded to Mamma's question, telling her that Papà had gone to the flea market with Rich.

"The flea *marketta?*" Mamma nearly whispered in disbelief. "*Con Rich?*"

I brushed by her and breezed my way into the kitchen. Mamma, still in her crumpled nightgown, followed. I buried my head inside the refrigerator.

"*Ma, perche?*" an annoyed Mamma asked "why" as she slumped into a seat at the kitchen table.

Although I was inclined to pose the same question to Papà, I wasn't as inclined to allow Mamma to do the same. "*Perche no?*" I responded as I emerged from the refrigerator, juggling eggs and butter for my breakfast—"Why not"? Then I followed up with an ask of what she would be doing all day.

Mamma turned her head away from me and set her stony sights on the water-spotted window. I watched as her black, watery eyes quickly glazed over and became hypnotized on absolute nothingness. She'd been so beautiful, once—her black tresses perfectly framing her milky-white face. I saw myself for just a moment back in time, watching Mamma as I sat on the potty. She'd comb her long, silky mane, then twist it and wrap it into a tight little bun at the nape of her neck. She'd then run that blood-red lipstick across her lips and blot it with a napkin before turning to wipe my bottom. On the outside, she looked oh-so-dramatic and oh-so-hard, as if touching her might chip her. On the inside, though, she was soft and gentle, like the Mamma she was meant to be.

But now, all color was gone. Sallow and sunken were her trademarks. Her once glorious hair had become a dingy gray, close-cropped mop, adding untold years to her sixty-year-old features. The only drama left in her now, if there was any still to be found, was whatever scene played out beneath the surface—under her skin and in her head—every time she zoned out or freaked out, depending on whether or not she was taking her meds.

She suddenly became aware of me watching her. She struggled to lift her long-fingered hands and limply, almost self-consciously, ran them through her hair.

"*Hai mangiato, Mamma?*"

She waved her hand at me, indicating she hadn't eaten.

I pulled out a frying pan from one of the cabinets to the left of the stove, placed it onto a burner, and lit the flame.

"*Uova? Café?*"

I asked if she wanted eggs or coffee as I plopped the butter into the skillet and watched it bubble. I cracked two eggs in as well, tossing the shells in the kitchen wastebasket, and tried to shake off my distaste for the shell of the woman who sat before me now. *Why did you have to get sick?* I turned my back to her as I continued to cook. I could feel her eyes upon me, but I refused to turn around and face her.

After a few heavy moments, Mamma replied in her usual, defeated voice. "*No, Paolettamia. Sono stanca. Mi vado ha fare un sonetto.*"

I nodded, still not turning to face her. She was tired and needed a nap, she said. I could hear her strain to rise, hear her feet in those tattered slippers she refused to toss out slowly shuffling out of the room, onto the carpeted hallway, and back to her bedroom.

That had been Mamma's routine since my return from ISU. I supposed it was better to have the sluggish Mamma than the rabid version.

Why can't we have one that's in between?

One who's normal?

I had no answer. As I stared at my two eggs, my only thoughts were of what Mamma's illness meant for me. Had I inherited her schizophrenic genes? Was crazy in my DNA? I took the spatula and started chopping up my breakfast. I had nine more years to wait and worry.

CHAPTER ELEVEN: **CONVENIENCE**

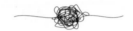

BACK-TO-SCHOOL COMMERCIALS on TV used to excite me. Every year growing up, new shoes for school, notebooks, pencils, and pens would make it to my shopping list. This year would be the first in two decades that that wouldn't be the case. I wouldn't be returning to school at all.

It would have been one thing if I had graduated college and was now going on to work in my chosen field of study, but that wasn't the case. I was in limbo, not yet done with my education and not yet able to finish. Now every time a back-to-school ad or flyer or conversation about school came my way, I felt left out and resentful.

It's your own damn fault.

Was it? Was it entirely my fault that I didn't have the finances to get my college degree?

You spent how much on out-of-state tuition?

How much credit card debt do you have?

Okay. So it was my fault. That part of it, anyway. But most normal families had the money or did the work to find it so that their kids could get a college education. I had to figure it out all by myself. And I had to help take care of things around here with Mamma and Viny. It just wasn't fair.

Having a pity party again?

Bitter, party for one?

It was tough when even I argued with me and ended up losing the battle. No matter how, I knew that I had to get my college degree, or I'd end up slaving away like poor Papà.

Caterina has a degree. She's not exactly whistling while she works.

Rosario is already working in architecture without a degree, and he's not slaving away.

Even Viny has a job and is going back to Pioneer Center for job skill services.

That was all true. But what was true for me? I didn't know. What I decided was best, at least for now, was to give myself another year to pay off my debt, apply to new schools, figure out how to fund the rest of my education, and basically get my act together.

You forgot lose weight and find a boyfriend.

They were right. I was right back where I'd started the year before. Nothing had changed. As a matter of fact, maybe it was worse. One step forward, two steps back.

I tried to model myself after Papà, but, obviously, I was failing. He had retired from his full-time job at the food processing plant, yet here he was, pushing seventy and working a part-time job to earn the extra money we needed. Now he supplemented his social security checks, earning the maximum allowed by the government, as a bagger at the grocery store Dominick's—not the one by the cemetery but one in nearby Crystal Lake.

Most people might have been ashamed of or felt demeaned by that job. Not Papà. He loved it. And the people at work loved him. Mothers with little children especially loved to have Papà—or Tony, as they called him—bag their groceries. It wasn't his skill as a bagger so much that had his checkout lines the longest (although he prided himself on being among the best and fastest); rather, it was how he took the time to entertain the little ones, innocently flirt with the moms and female checkers, and joke with the guys, making them all feel special.

That was one of Papà's gifts. He found joy in everything he did, and he brought joy to others just by being himself.

One day, after returning from work, he excitedly recounted how the Kellogg's Frosted Flakes mascot had visited the grocery store. The famous orange and black cat with the bandana around his neck had all of the children clamoring to take pictures with him.

Papà said he asked his coworkers, "Who he be?" Upon learning it was Tony the Tiger, he'd marched right up to him, determined to shake the tiger's hand. It wasn't that Papà was somehow star struck over some product spokesperson. It was because they bore the same name, and that gave Papà an opportunity to share one of his favorite jokes.

Licking his lips, trying to master his imperfect English, he'd done his best to get his point across: "You name be Tony? Maybe you be *Italiano* too, *si*? Know why so many *Italianos* be name Tony?"

Papà took out a piece of paper and wrote on it, then held it up for the tiger to see.

"This be what show they when go off boat. To Newa York. See? TONY. My name Tony, too. Nice meet you."

Tony the Tiger roared, Papà said. Everyone else laughed too, the loudest being Papà himself, who posed with the tiger for a picture.

I learned from picking Papá up after work—from the checkers who told me they called themselves his girlfriends and who loved when Papà called them "my dollies" and from the mothers who insisted on bringing their children and checking out in the lane he was bagging for that day—that Papà was more popular than even that tiger with everyone at the store.

For Halloween that year, Papà told me that everyone at Dominick's was supposed to come to work dressed up in costume. He waved his hand and scrunched up his face, pretending not to care.

"Sono troppo vecchio."

"You're not too old, Papà," I responded. Then, before I thought it through, I heard myself committing to making him a Halloween costume.

You should be committed.

You don't have time for that.

Mamma's the one who knows how to sew.

No, I didn't really have time. But Mamma wasn't in any condition to help. She had her own challenges, including even remembering to shower on most days. She still believed that cameras inside the home were photographing her whenever she was nude, so bathing posed a real problem for her. Her refusal to consistently take her meds meant that we never knew for sure if today was the day she would take her revenge out on the people she thought were trying to kill her—us—or if we were safe for one more day.

Nothing could shake Mamma's belief that the doctors were experimenting on her. It was her reasoning for why she hadn't yet been cured of her illness. On her worst days, usually when she had to be taken for one of her doctor's appointments, she would scream and yell and try to scratch Papà, believing he was working in cahoots with whoever was in charge of her demise.

For some reason even I didn't understand, committing to making a Halloween costume for Papà was a must for me. I think I saw it as an opportunity to distract Mamma from the madness. She loved to sew. I hadn't a clue how to. Together, maybe we could succeed in making something that would bring everybody a little bit of joy.

When buying the dark brown and white felt material from the fabric store, I figured it wouldn't be that difficult to turn Papà into a larger-than-life package of M&M'S chocolate candies. After all, it was just a front and a back and some lettering and then cinching the top and bottom so that they looked like tiny ruffles, sort of how the actual individual packs did. Surely, I could do this with Mamma's help.

But Mamma wasn't too keen on helping. So instead, I ended up spending hours upon hours, every morning before heading to work and every evening upon returning home, crafting Papà's Halloween costume. Mamma occasionally hovered over me, silently monitoring my progress and offering up suggestions that felt more like criticisms, but she never once picked up a needle and thread.

If necessity was the mother of invention, expectations were the mother of frustration. And I seemed to be the "mother" experiencing both with this costume.

I'd bought bags of actual M&M's, planning to use them to accurately trace the logo's lettering on the real packaging. I hadn't exactly thought through how to turn something no bigger than the size of my palm into something big enough to be displayed on the length of Papà's body. In the end, I did my best to freehand the infamous "m" on a large enough scale so it would look decent at life-size—and I actually think I succeeded.

Shock of shocks, so did Mamma.

"*Brava!*" She exclaimed upon seeing my handiwork. I couldn't help but smile at what seemed like genuine praise.

Her encouragement had me thinking I could make pockets for Papà and stuff them with the real candy so he could reach inside himself, so to speak, and hand out M&M's to the children at the grocery store on Halloween.

Great idea, but the execution fell short. Days later, when I finished the costume, the new plan became for Papà to wear shorts that had lots of pockets underneath the giant homemade costume. We then stuffed the pockets of his shorts with child-sized packets of the candy for him to hand out.

One final accessory: a white little beret made out of felt that he wore as a hat, covering his bald head. It, too, had the M&M logo on top.

It was the best I could do.

And it turned out to be enough.

Papà and his M&M's costume were a huge hit. All the moms and kids waited to go through Tony's checkout so that they could get a hug from Mr. M&M and some candy, too. Papà said that every time he hiked up his costume to reach into his pockets to get the packets of candy for the children, his "girlfriends," who worked as other baggers and cashiers, whistled in appreciation of his legs. Papà giggled like a little kid.

MAMMA, ON THE OTHER HAND, wasn't so amused. She had now gotten it into her head that Papà had real girlfriends, and that this was just another reason why he no longer showed her much affection.

Off her meds, Mamma ranted and threatened and screamed nonsense, often through the night. On her meds, she wavered between totally catatonic and unaware and being some sort of ghost—the kind that snuck up on you and stared you down accusingly for something you had no idea you'd done. Because you hadn't. It was all in her head.

The trick I kept needing to master was to not let it get into my head. To that end, I did my best to pretend that neither extreme of Mamma really existed.

The madness at home kept me up at night. I listened for every little sound that might signify danger: the click-click of the stove's burners igniting; Mamma's whispers to no one as she paced the living room, making the floorboards creak; the garage door opening and closing for no good reason; Papà's snoring and me paying attention to make sure it did not stop (proof that he was still breathing).

Lack of sleep and constant worry caused my focus at my job to suffer. Still learning the nuts and bolts of what to do, I couldn't seem to do it fast enough for my supervisor. Numbers weren't my thing, words were. When I tried to balance the figures on the spreadsheets, I always came up with errors.

One day, when everyone else who had finished their tallies had already left for lunch, I wasn't allowed to. Until I succeeded in balancing my numbers down to the penny, I wouldn't be dismissed for break.

I tried and tried to figure out the missing pennies on my own. I just couldn't do it. The boss saw me continuing to struggle and walked over to me. She had bank deposits and other things to do, each with their own deadlines, and she couldn't do any of them until I submitted my dailies to her.

Looking over my work, she shook her head in disapproval. "Go," she snipped at me.

"I can do it again," I stammered, near to tears.

"Just go!" she ordered. She grabbed my work from my desk and carried it off to her own to finish what I could not.

The staff breakroom wasn't much more than a kitchenette with a table and some plastic chairs. I stood near the sink, staring down at the countertop. I felt like such a failure. *Why can't I do this job? What if I'm not smart enough to do any job? What if I get fired? How will I ever make enough money to go back to school? How will I pay my credit card bills? I'll be stuck at home forever.*

My boss had followed me into the room, but I hadn't noticed. I had become a zombie. When I finally heard her calling my name, I couldn't help but start bawling like a baby.

"Hey," she said, her eyebrows raised and her entire expression filled with concern. "It's okay. It's just a spreadsheet. I found where you were off."

I shook my head. I was inconsolable. I didn't hear anything else she said, and I couldn't stop sobbing. She quickly took hold of me and ushered me into her office. Sitting me down, she sat beside me in silence—and somehow, without meaning to, I told her about Mamma and the madness at home.

As good as it felt to spill my secret to her, I immediately regretted having done so. I had never wanted to be seen as anything other than a success, a powerhouse, the smart one, the one who had her shit together. I wasn't clinically insane like Mamma. And I wasn't someone who needed extra help like Viny. I made sure to apologize for my meltdown and assured my supervisor that it would never happen again. I also made her promise to never bring up or share what I had told her with me or anybody else. She agreed to keep my secret.

AFTER WORK, I DROVE HOME.

Once I arrived, I didn't want to go into the house. I didn't trust myself alone with Mamma or Viny. Sometimes, I would eat just to shut my mouth. I feared I would say things to them that I couldn't take back. Even worse, I sometimes wished Mamma dead and for Viny to just disappear.

I sat on the front steps of our home, my fist holding up my chin. My head felt so heavy. I wished Mr. A was sitting next to me, making me laugh.

INSTEAD, PAPÀ'S SILVER PONTIAC rambled down our street and turned into our driveway. My eyes followed, connecting with his through the passenger window. I could read it on his face: worry, probably because of what he must be seeing in mine.

He pushed the button on the remote that hung on his car's visor, opening the garage door so that he could drive in. When he parked the car inside, he came out to greet me.

"*La bimba che aspetta,*" he said.

I sighed, my head still balancing on my fist. I was too old to be called a child, I thought. But I was, indeed, waiting. For what, exactly, even I didn't know. And Papà didn't ask. He sat down next to me on the concrete step and began reciting from memory, his hands gesturing with every phrase: "'*Che fai bambina mia su quella porta, guardando da lontan per quella via?' Ah, sapessi, quando la fu morta, se la portaron via di là la mamma mia, e mi hanno detto che di là deve tornare, e son quì da tanti anni ad aspettare!*'"

Papà always amazed me at the poetry he could recite without a single misstep of words or failure in memory.

I listened as he brought the poem to life, softly asking the child what she was doing, gazing off into the distance? The child explained that her mamma was taken away because she died, and they told her that she would return from where they had taken her. So now "*la bimba*" waited. My papà's tone deepened further as he struggled to finish, the lump in his throat growing.

"'*Cara bambina mia ma tu non sai, che i morti al mondo non ritornano mai?*'"

The passerby asks, "Dear little child of mine, don't you know that the dead don't ever return to this world?"

"*Tornano nel vaso i fiorellini miei, tornan le stelle, tornerà anche lei!*"

The child responds that the flowers in her vase grow back, the stars come back at night, and so, too, will her mamma.

This was why she waited, explained Papà.

"*Che aspetti tu, bimba mia?*" he asked.

What was I waiting for? I wasn't sure I knew. "*Niente, Papà.*" Again, I said, "Nothing."

Papà then explained that the little girl in the poem, which he had learned long ago, was also named Paolina, and that she eventually turned to marble after waiting so many days and nights in the cold for her dead mother to return home. When he drove up, he said, he saw in me that little girl, someone he never wanted me to be.

A marble statue waiting: I didn't want to be that either. But I felt as if I was always waiting and never quite getting—either what I wanted or where I wanted to be. I certainly wasn't waiting for Mamma, the version I loved, to return, for I had given up on that hope. No, I guess I was waiting for my life to begin—the part with less of the madness and more of whatever was on the other side of crazy. I was waiting for normal. Waiting for that thing that felt to me like some elusive magic. But was it too late for me? Had my heart and soul grown cold? Had I already turned to stone?

CHAPTER TWELVE: **CHAOS**

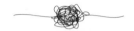

ATTENDING COMMUNITY COLLEGE FOR a couple of years to knock out undergraduate requirements and save money and then transferring to a university of choice is a pretty smart strategy for earning a degree. My path was anything but.

Northern Illinois University in DeKalb, about thirty-five miles southwest of Algonquin, accepted me for the fall 1987 semester. Since I already finished three years at other schools—two at University of Illinois at Chicago and the year before last at Iowa State University—I should have been a senior, but I didn't have enough credits for the right classes. So I transferred in as a junior.

We told you so.

Horseback riding, what a stupid move.

I had to quit my full-time job and find a part-time job that paid well enough for me to finish school. Because I needed to work as many hours as possible, that meant I had to be at school as few days as possible. It was a balancing act I wasn't sure I could pull off. The minimum number of days on campus would be two: Tuesdays and Thursdays. Those didn't leave too many course options that satisfied graduation requirements. I settled for Intro to Mathematics, Intro to Visual Arts, and Intro to Social Psychology.

How can you be classified as a junior and still be taking introductory courses?

A great question for which I had no answer. Unlike my classes at ISU, where I'd felt such excitement being in them no matter what the subject, the courses at NIU were all a means to the most normal end: graduation, a real paying job, and living out on my own.

I needed to find one more class to fill my twelve-credit class requirement to be considered a full-time student. The only other class still open that fit my Tuesday/Thursday requirement, and that I was remotely interested in, was something called Exceptional Persons in Society. I thought it was a class about heroes or people doing great things; turned out, it wasn't. It actually fell under the Learning, Development, and Special Education Department. In reading its description, the one person who came to my mind was Viny, and the possibility of equating Viny's "not normal" with her being "exceptional" drew me in.

Now all I needed was to find the actual job to pay for school.

I lined up three interviews for three different jobs. One was as the "information girl" at Spring Hill Mall. It paid $4.50 per hour. The second was for a medical assistant to a pediatrician. It paid $5.00 per hour. The third was a temporary job for the Ace Pecan Company, a Christmas catalog kind of place that sold nuts and candy. The work was mindless data entry every Monday, Wednesday, Friday, and weekends, and it paid $6.50 per hour. It also offered as much overtime as I could handle.

I was offered all of them, and it was a no-brainer which one I took.

School became mindless, too. Commuting versus living on campus translated into me never quite being "all in" with either my subjects or my classmates. I was one foot into academia and one foot into the working world, and I didn't really care for either. What I did care for, I no longer could have. I missed Beth and Kathy and Shelly and Dr. Mack and Professor Hadley and Janet and Marie and both of my Charlies.

I missed, most of all, me.

THE TEACHER OF MY EXCEPTIONAL Persons in Society class talked a lot about fitting in. And yet Dr. Elliott Lessen, with his homegrown, boyish looks, Ralph Lauren dress shirts, and snappy personality, made it clear that he didn't much care about fitting in.

"No two people are exactly alike," he said as he eased his way throughout the classroom. He went on to explain that people with disabilities were, just like everybody else, unique individuals. He made a great point: just because someone had a disability in one area didn't mean they were disabled in all areas.

And then he asked us if we could think of someone we knew who had a disability.

Nothing to see here.

While Mamma came to mind, as did Viny, I knew better than to disclose my family's secrets.

The students who did respond shared about cerebral palsy, blindness, hearing impairments—they all focused more on physical sorts of disabilities. I perked up when the conversation wound its way around to what Dr. Lessen referred to as chronic problems involving the brain. Someone talked about epilepsy, calling it "mysterious" and a family crisis. Shame, guilt, blame, fear—these were the words they used, the very same ones that plagued me.

Feeling helpless because of an inability to control or fix the problem, Dr. Lessen said, often led to overprotectiveness on the part of parents or caregivers in these types of cases.

I slowly nodded, realizing that the same sort of thing was happening with Viny. While she didn't have epilepsy, something wasn't right with her.

"*Era come se fosse caduta dal cielo, e la terra l'ha cresciuta,*" Papà would say.

Literally, it translated to, "It was as if she dropped from the sky, and the earth grew her." Figuratively, it meant that she was a mystery who aged but who failed to learn or retain what life had to teach her. She couldn't take care of herself, and yet she didn't have enough brain power, it seemed, to understand or even acknowledge that fact. So she rebelled.

The more Viny pushed for her independence, the more her freedoms were restricted. Screaming fits between her and Papà had by now become weekly events. It often felt as if we were ringside at one of Iron Mike Tyson's boxing matches. Papà loved the sport and this fighter who almost always won with a knockout. Sometimes, I wished he would throw a punch to knock out Viny and shut her up.

When Dr. Lessen's class turned more toward emotional and behavioral disorders, I felt as if I should have brought in Viny for show-and-tell, just like the ISU no-name hawk. It was one thing to read about disabilities and theorize about what they did or didn't mean; it was a very different ballgame when it was part of your reality. Viny had always struggled academically, from the time she started school. She also had social and emotional problems.

In high school at Niles North in Skokie, the school hadn't known or hadn't cared about what they should do with Viny. Rather than get her the help she needed, they'd lumped her into a class for emotionally and behaviorally disruptive students. At the time, Viny had been neither—and in that class, she'd been afraid to speak or catch any kid's eye. The abuse and bullying she'd suffered at the hands of other students—and not just those in that particular class—had been criminal.

One day, Viny came home with a hole in her hand—a pencil stab, courtesy of one of her many abusers. Rosario became so enraged that he accompanied her to school the next day, walked right inside with her, and asked her to point out the boy who had been hurting her. She did, and Rosario proceeded to grab the kid, throw him into the lockers, pin him there, and threaten to do some major bodily harm to him if he or anyone else even looked at Viny sideways ever again.

That succeeded in putting an end to the physical bullying. Rosario received a stern warning from the school and authorities, but he welcomed it. He turned the tables on them, exposing their lack of security measures and threatening to come back if they didn't do their jobs and stop the bullying.

All her life, Viny had stuck to the shadows to avoid getting noticed, at school and at home. But lately, things were different. Her return to those McHenry County Social Services and Pioneer Center programs seemed to be helping her come out of her shell more. She spent time with friends now, and that right there was a pretty major accomplishment, since she'd never really had any friends before. She was also learning basic life skills, like budgeting and cooking.

The changes in Viny's behavior were definitely noticeable and good in so many ways, but something inside me wondered if they were going too far and doing just as much harm as good—if not more harm than good. She was embracing their teachings about self-empowerment, but she was taking it to the extreme. The rise in her confidence and socializing didn't take into account her impaired thought processes and cognitive abilities. It was as if they had given a child a cape and a mask and told her she could fly, only to have her jump off a rooftop and fall to her death as a result. That was a problem.

She's not your kid.

She ain't your problem.

True. Viny wasn't mine to worry about. I shook off all thoughts of her. My only concern should be getting out of school, leaving my family's legacy behind, and finally living a life on my own.

PROBLEM WAS, I STILL NEEDED to figure out what that life might be. And time was up for me—at least, according to NIU's policies.

By the time I had sixty semester hours under my belt, I was supposed to have declared a major. I was late, again, already having accumulated more than eighty. The major that made the most sense for me was a bachelor's in communication with an emphasis in media studies. And even if I went that route, in order to graduate by May of 1989 – two years beyond when I should have graduated – I had to shift from attending classes just two days per week to being on campus all five days.

That was a problem. It required a new job, one that would allow me to work late nights and/or on Saturdays and Sundays. While that would mean that I would be committed pretty much 24/7 to either school or work, it was the only way for me to reach my goals and pay for it all.

The job at Ace Pecan ended just after Christmas that year. It had only been a temporary gig anyway. I hunted for something else to bring in the dollars and found the perfect match. By February of 1988, my twenty-third birthday, I was working weekends for a builder of luxury homes. I had no interest in construction or real estate, but the job offered the hours and the pay I needed. And it also gave me something else: autonomy.

The little, single-story, cottage-like home that doubled as the company's headquarters sat all on its own along a busy stretch of road just a few blocks from the Barrington train station. The office had to have been someone's home at one time. Now it stood isolated, with nothing else around it. Barely any customers visited or even phoned in for information, at least not on the weekends—and I didn't work on weekdays.

What I loved most about the job was the solitude. Being on my own from 9:00 a.m. until 4:00 p.m. every Saturday and Sunday translated into peace and quiet, the very opposite of what went on at home. And I spent every moment sitting at the front desk, dreaming up what my life would be, doing my schoolwork, and writing my stories.

With my senior status at school, all of my classes included some aspect of creative writing. Storyboarding and writing television commercials, writing and recording radio spots, actually working in a television studio to produce student shows—I loved every second of it. But the one class I loved the most was screenwriting.

Something inside me came alive at the thought of writing not just short stories, as I had done with Professor Hadley at ISU, but scripts. I always had loved films, and the thought of my words being brought to life with graphics and movie sets and actors, and then having audiences applauding my stories as the credits rolled on *my* movie on the theater's big screen . . .

I daydreamed of the Oscar speech I would give: "I'd like to thank the Academy . . ."

Seriously?

You haven't even written your first screenplay.

They mocked my acceptance speech rehearsals. But I didn't. On my ninety-minute drives to and from school, I practiced. And I gave the voices in my head, my constant companions, something to do, too, assigning them roles as different characters in my stories.

MIDWAY THROUGH THE SEMESTER IN one of my media writing classes, we were asked to analyze a TV comedy or drama. A new TV series, *Beauty and the Beast*, had recently debuted. In it, a Shakespeare-quoting half man/half beast and a wealthy socialite attorney crossed paths and joined forces to battle crime, and they slowly fell for one another. It became my obsession, as did the study of the relationship between beauty and beast, prey and predator, the good and evil that exists in the outside world and that lives within us all.

I hoped that what spoke to me was really normal versus the start of the demons that waited to rise from within. Maybe I hadn't done enough to make sure Mamma's madness stayed clear of me. I still had years to go before turning thirty, that magical age when I could breathe, knowing I had escaped Mamma's mental illness genes. Yet, part of me still feared that somewhere, in some other part of me, the voices, the hallucinations, the paranoia, the legacy lurked.

I focused on the series, studying not just the story elements and the production aspects but also the character profiles. The assumption of such darkness in the Beast and such light in the Beauty proved false in the television show; neither one of them was all good or all evil. Maybe those assumptions would prove just as false in real life, even mine.

In my screenwriting class, I learned about writing "on spec"—basically, writing something without any promise of anyone ever buying it. A spec script's purpose was to showcase the writer's talents enough to get her a paying gig, though in a best-case scenario it might be sold and produced. No guarantees, of course, but big money could be made if it did sell. *Lethal Weapon*, the buddy cop movie that had recently been released, had been written by a twenty-three-year-old guy. *The very same age as me*, I thought. It was his first spec script, and it had sold for a quarter of a million dollars.

Could we do that?

Why not? I set out to write an original episode of *Beauty and the Beast* on spec. It wasn't just the money that tempted me; rather, it was the storytelling, the magic of making movies, and the dream of one day giving my well-rehearsed acceptance speech on stage in Hollywood.

THAT FIRST SCRIPT I SUBMITTED for the TV series got me an invitation to send it to the William Morris Talent Agency. I had no idea who Arthur Dreifuss was or how he had gotten my name, but I didn't hesitate to follow through. Neither did I stop there. Suddenly, scripts started pouring out of me. The next two I wrote on spec were full-length feature screenplays: *Tarzan and Jane*, an opposites-attract romantic comedy, and *Darker Sides*, a good-guy-gone-bad thriller.

I wrote and wrote and submitted to competitions and internships in Los Angeles. I now had my sights set on becoming a screenwriter and moving to the West Coast.

Even Lee from ISU wrote a recommendation on my behalf for an internship at the Academy of Television Arts and Sciences.

If part of your reputation rests, as does Iowa State University's, on what students produce in future years, you have a winner in Paolina Milana. I'd stake my teaching and writing career on that.

If I can be of any further help, please let me know.

Sincerely,

Lee Hadley
Associate Professor of English

Lee said she'd stake her career on me being a winner; so would I, I thought. I was so sure I would get in. And I couldn't wait to tell Professor Hadley that I had not only gotten accepted to the program but had, of course, sold all my spec scripts. She would definitely get an invitation to my Oscar party! I'd fly her out and put her in the grandest hotel!

But instead of getting accepted, what came in the mail were rejections from every competition, internship, and talent agency I had submitted to. Dozens of form letters that I didn't bother to read beyond the first few lines arrived, each one greeting me with, "Dear Writer: Although you were not chosen . . ." A postcard also came in the mail from Arthur Dreifuss at the William Carroll Agency, advising me that I'd be receiving all of what I had sent to him unopened. According to the typed note, a "defunct agency without our consent" was at fault for the crossed wires. However they worded their messages, it was clear: I wasn't wanted, and my writing wasn't good enough to even warrant a review.

Who do you think you are?

Professor Hadley softened the blow, starting off her letter with, *"Dear Paolina: Rats!"* That, alone, made me giggle. The rest of her letter, however, made me think:

In other words, you didn't do anything wrong. You might well have been competing with people who already had writing credits. And, believe it or not, you do have what you want/need--you have ambition, drive, talent and desire--just don't get side-tracked and settle for second best; after all, you're on your way to being one of the best.

I took her words to heart and kept writing whenever I could, devoting as much of my Saturdays and Sundays working on my own stories as I could, including while I was at work. And every weekday morning, I'd leave the house before the sun rose, mostly to beat the traffic on my way to school but also to work on stories and school assignments before actual classes consumed my days. Mandatory lab hours to learn how to work all of the equipment and positions in TV production added to my load. By the time I headed back home, darkness surrounded me, and rarely would I see another car on the road.

ONE NIGHT, A WINTER STORM dumped so much snow on the country road I traveled that it turned it from a two-lane into a lane-and-a-half, at best, before my drive home. And with the snow drifts scattered here and there, parts of the road were nearly impassable.

I never feared my solo drives to and from school, but on this particular night, I did. The radio kept me company, making me feel less alone. At one point, my heater didn't seem to be working in my little Ford Escort, so I found myself alternating between wiping clear enough of a circle on the fogged-up windshield so I could see through it and rubbing my hands together so they wouldn't freeze.

I could barely make out the headlights pointed in my direction in the distance. In what seemed like just moments later, those high beams were barreling toward me. While I could clearly see the snow plow dead ahead, he didn't seem aware of me at all. Despite flashing my headlights, the plow driver wasn't moving over. I had no choice but to swerve out of his way—landing my car in a ditch.

This would make a great scene in some story.

Only if we caught up to that driver and murdered him.

Murder. I agreed, exhaling in frustration. A simple solution to a lot of problems. If only I could guarantee I wouldn't get caught. My shaky hands turned off the motor, not wanting to add running out of gas to my dilemma. Unhurt, but with no clue how to get out of where I was stuck, I sat for a few moments in the silence. As I looked outside at the snow-covered countryside surrounding me, I suddenly erupted in laughter that quickly gave way to bawling.

I didn't know if the snow plow driver really hadn't seen me or if he was a psycho who wondered what it would be like to run someone off the road, maybe even killing them. No one would even know if he'd intended to leave a body behind in the car crash he'd caused. Maybe he was going to circle back and finish the job.

You need to get out of here.

You are so losing it.

I was shifting between sobbing and giggling; my imagination was getting the best of me. Hopefully, it wasn't anything more. Oh, the irony of "going off the deep end" while being stuck in a ditch!

Lee's words echoed in my head: *Don't get side-tracked.*

I straightened up in my seat, wiped away my tears, turned the key in the ignition, and once again started the engine. Papà had made sure to put a little shovel and old cardboard boxes in the back of my hatchback. I hadn't been sure what for when he did it, but now I had a need, and they were all I had to make my way out of the hole I had fallen into.

I exited my car, opened up the back, took out my tools, and began to alternate between digging behind the back wheels, shoving cardboard underneath them, getting back in the car, pressing on the gas and rocking my Escort back and forth and back and forth, and repeating the process again, until finally, I set my car free and got it back up onto the road.

The ordeal had taken me at least an hour, if not more. I was sure that when I entered into my home, Papà would be waiting up, so worried. Maybe even Mamma would be with him. I could only imagine what they must be thinking, with me not getting home at my usual time. I hoped they hadn't called the police or anything.

My envisioning of the missing persons' drama unfolding at home fizzled out as soon as I climbed the steps from the garage to the living room and realized that everybody had already gone to bed. They hadn't even left a night light on for me. It was completely dark. Did they even think of what I might have encountered? Did I even matter to them? To anyone? Even Papà?

I climbed into bed, quietly crying.

Viny, from her bunk up above, softly called out, "What's the matter, Pauley?"

I swallowed back my tears. "Nothing, Vince. Go back to bed. It's nothing."

IN THE SPRING OF THAT YEAR—May 20, 1988, to be exact—I stood in my living room, staring at the TV, mesmerized by the unfolding news of a woman named Laurie Dann who had just shot six children in a nearby elementary school just miles from my house. The stand-off with police would end with her committing suicide. Those interviewed detailed a long history of societal withdrawal, erratic behavior, and psychological intervention, but said no one could have predicted the tragedy.

I couldn't help the involuntary nodding of my head. As people blamed family, friends, and authorities for not doing more sooner, I couldn't help but think, *There but for the grace of God go I.*

As the debate over committing people with mental illnesses, who were incapable of making informed decisions about their own care, to health facilities against their will ignited, I knew that most of those who were talking about it really hadn't a clue. And those of us who did were scared to share our truth. Mamma proved the point that it didn't really matter if you did have someone committed, because it was a temporary solution to a never-ending problem. It wasn't as if you could keep people committed forever. At some point, ready or not, they had to be released. And then the whole cycle of going off meds and getting hospitalized would repeat.

To think of mental illness as some broken bone—something easily seen, identified, and treatable to the point of being cured—was the actual insanity.

I needed to finish school, get my degree, get out of the madness that was my family, and get on with my own life.

CHAPTER THIRTEEN: **CROSSROADS**

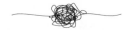

THAT FINAL YEAR BLURRED BY, not just because of my own school and work but because we were planning for a wedding. Caterina had finally met a guy who had turned out to be "the one." No longer would she consider herself a member of our Valentine's Day lonely hearts club; she would marry in October of 1988.

By that time, Rosario was rarely around. He had moved into his own apartment in one of downtown Chicago's up-and-coming River North high-rises, right next to the Merchandise Mart where he worked.

Both he and Caterina had escaped.

At least Viny and I no longer had to share the same room. She took over Caterina's bedroom, taking her top bunk with her. I still slept on my bottom bunk, but for the first time in what totaled four years, I did so staring up at a ceiling instead of up at the underside of a snoring someone else. I relished the silence. My room was the one place I had that was my own. I could escape there and pretend it was just me.

Mamma had gone off her meds again. With every cycle of taking drugs that controlled her and then stopping and going completely out of control, she worsened. Longer hospital stays, prescription cocktails that no longer worked, periods of rage and accusations, and then a new drug recipe that led to a mummified existence.

The time had come: Papà needed to escape.

His childhood friend from Sicily had for decades been living in San Diego. He was invited to visit for a long weekend. He asked my permission to go. Could I handle Mamma on my own?

I so wanted to say no, please don't leave me. But it was only for a few days. And he needed a break. Understanding that, I figured I could deal with Mamma.

Mamma immediately proved me wrong.

Papà's friend was female, and that sent a paranoid Mamma into a downward spiral. She telephoned him constantly the first day of his trip, ranting, threatening that if he didn't come home that very second, she'd hurt us.

Papà raced back.

This was his fate.

I couldn't let it be mine.

FINALLY, ON MAY 13, 1989, after six long years of work, I succeeded in walking across the stage at NIU, shaking the university president's hand, and collecting my diploma.

Now what?

Great question. I hadn't a clue. I had been so busy dealing with the madness at home, working, and just trying to get through school that I'd forgotten about the career I was in school to actually get. Frantically, I began applying to whatever I could find in the local newspapers.

"*Non ti preocupare, Paolamia,*" Papà consoled me as he gently caressed the cluster of white grapes growing on one of his vines. "*Ci dissi u surci a nuci; dammi tempu ca ti perciu.*"

I wanted to not worry. I even understood what Papà meant by yet another of his favorite proverbs: "The mouse said to the nut: give me time and I shall reach you." But patience had never been my strong suit, even if persistence was.

As Papà meticulously pruned, focusing his energies on raising his miracle babies, I watched and wondered at his green thumb. How could anyone magically grow these ancient vines here in the Midwest, where they had little chance of even taking root, let alone thriving? These beautiful baubles of fruit, their translucent skin sparkling in the sunlight, proved that anything was possible if you were willing to love it into existence.

I asked Papà if this would be the year his grapes would be ready to be picked and turned into wine.

He shook his head and winked at me, a huge grin on his face. "*L'anno prossimo che vieni,*" he replied. "*Non sono ancora abbastanza maturi o dolci—come te.*"

The grapes would be ready to harvest next year. They weren't mature or sweet—like me—yet, he said. I rolled my eyes.

Sweet?

Not!

What would your Papà say if he knew the real you?

Beauty and beast, prey and predator, good and evil—the screenplays I had written, even if they weren't good enough to get me signed, all told my story, focusing on the battle within. The TV shows and movies I loved to watch all had characters with both a dark and a light side. But that was normal . . . wasn't it? Even Papà had once told me, "*A volte, bisogna farli vedere i denti.*" Translation: *Sometimes, you need to show them your teeth.*

I had grown somewhat fearful of mine.

TWO MONTHS AFTER GRADUATING AND into my job hunt, I finally ran across a tiny blind ad in the daily newspaper classifieds for a copywriter. It didn't include much more than "writer wanted" in terms of what the job was all about. It didn't even give the name of the company that had placed the ad. I didn't care, as long as the word "writer" was the job being offered.

During that time, I also wrote a letter to Oprah Winfrey.

Who do you think you are?

Her show taped at Harpo Productions in Chicago, and it had become a daily "must-see" for me. Even Mamma would sit with me to watch. Viny rarely did; she chose to sleep in or stay locked in her room. I asked in my letter to become a member of Oprah's team. I knew getting any kind of response from Oprah or anyone at Harpo was a long shot, but I also knew that if I didn't try, there was a 100 percent guarantee of it never happening.

THE COMPANY THAT HAD PLACED the blind classified ad called me in to interview for the job. I couldn't believe it. The job was for the third largest newspaper in Illinois called the *Daily Herald*. Me? Working at a newspaper! I couldn't wait to tell Professor Hadley.

Focus! Ace the interview, or that can't happen.

As I sat in a windowless room barely bigger than a closet, its white walls devoid of any decoration, with nothing but the chair beneath me, the table in front of me, and a packet of papers with a pen waiting on top, I should have been nervous. But I wasn't.

This wasn't just an interview; it was a final exam, one that had the power to make or break me. I dove in. With every test the recruiter put in front of me—four hours' worth of word recognition, definitions, grammar, and timed assignments that instructed candidates to look at supplied photographs from which we were to craft captions and stories with specific character counts—I grew more and more excited. This was my chance to get closer to my dream of making a living as a writer.

What happened to California?

I thought you wanted to be a screenwriter?

California and screenwriting still called to me, but that bigger dream of leaving home, trekking cross-country, writing a feature film, and walking the red carpet would have to wait. I needed a job, and here in front of me was a real job willing to pay me to write.

Walking out of that interview, I confidently told everybody—friends, family, Papà's coworkers at the grocery store, anyone who would listen or happened to cross my path that day—that I had aced it. There wasn't a single doubt in my mind that I would be offered the job.

DAYS LATER, THE PHONE RANG. I picked it up.

"Hi, Paolina, this is Sharon in Human Resources from the *Daily Herald*."

"Yes!" I said, trying to contain my excitement, thinking this would be it.

"I'm sorry, but we're not going to be asking you back for this position."

What?

Sharon continued talking, but I had stopped listening. She had knocked the wind out of me, as surely as if she had punched me in the stomach. I fought to hold back the tears that immediately welled up in my eyes. When she paused long enough for me to realize she had finished, all I could manage to get out was a whimper, "Okay, thank you for letting me know."

I hung up the receiver, and immediately burst into tears. I had taken the call from the phone in my parents' bedroom and now I slumped down onto their bed, burying my face in my two hands to muffle my crying.

I hadn't gotten the job.

You told all those people you were a shoe-in.

How embarrassing.

How could you have been so wrong?

You must have really sucked.

Now what?

Before I could really think on my own, the phone rang again. I waited to hear if anyone else in the house would pick up, but they didn't, so I did.

"Hello?" I squeaked.

"Paolina, oh my gosh, it's Sharon again," the breathy voice on the other end of the line raced to say. "I'm so sorry. I made a mistake. I had two lists of candidates to call, and I got them mixed up. You're on the list we *want* to have come back in. Are you interested?"

Is she kidding?

My entire being flopped a bit, like pasta al dente. The air I had not even realized I was holding in rushed out as I tearfully blubbered, "Yes. Thank you. Yes."

While it would take a couple more interviews to make it official, in August of 1989, I succeeded in landing a job working as a paid copywriter at the suburban Chicago newspaper called the *Daily Herald*.

ON MY FIRST MORNING REPORTING to work, Papà made me breakfast as I got ready, as he usually did. I had spent hours on my hair, makeup, and dressing up in a brand-new blue and white skirt and blouse with matching shoes and accessories. The ladies at my old bridal registry job had gifted me with a leather briefcase that held my notebook and pens.

"*Li mangerai!*" Papà beamed, telling me again that I would eat them up!

Who he thought I'd be eating up, I wasn't quite sure, but I giggled at his faith in me and knew for sure that I looked smart. I felt like I was finally on my way. To where, exactly, I wasn't sure, but I knew this would lead me somewhere, and definitely out of where I was.

By this time next year, I promised myself, I, too, would move out. I started dreaming of my own place, maybe even in California; of having friends over; and of taking a bath in my own tub.

Driving in my Escort with the sunroof open on my way to the *Daily Herald* offices that day, I couldn't wait to get there.

I had left the house early and arrived early. Too early. Not wanting to seem over-eager, I doubled back to the gas station I had seen on my way in, figuring I would fill up my tank. I pulled into the self-serve, exited my car, unscrewed the gas tank cap, and pulled on the flexible hose that led down from the dispenser. Turning it on, I lifted the pump's nozzle and moved to insert it into my tank.

It took me a second to realize that the wet stuff dousing me was gasoline and was shooting out of the nozzle I was holding. By the time I turned off the pump, my new dress, my shoes, my hair, pretty much all of me had gotten sprayed, if not soaked.

The people at the other pumps barely seemed to notice. I hoped no one would light a match, or for sure, I would burst into flames. I stood frozen, unsure of what to do, until the manager came out of the station toward me, a look of shock on his face. He took the nozzle I still held, apologizing. Upon inspection, we both realized that someone had taped down the handle, causing gas to spew uncontrollably the second the pump got turned on.

Who would do that?

A conspiracy to keep you from starting your new job?

I didn't have time to dwell on it. And I sure didn't have time to head back home to change. The filling station manager helped me cover as much of my car's front seat as possible with paper towels, protecting it from my soiled clothes. He helped me dry off, too, and then filled my tank and let me drive off without paying.

Back at the newspaper's offices with not a minute to spare, I marched my dampened self, both in body and spirit, into the lobby. I tried my best to act normal, although I had no idea how a normal person who had just been doused with gasoline would behave. I explained to the main receptionist, who couldn't help but wrinkle her nose at the smell of me, that I was reporting for orientation. She nodded, trying to smile, and placed a call, alerting someone that I had arrived.

Within moments, my new boss, Karin, greeted me. She didn't seem to notice the condition I was in—or if she did, she didn't let on. With an outstretched hand, she welcomed me. Her eyes sparkled, and her smile lit up the room. She looked like what I imagined the mom of a cherub might resemble, if angels were to have their own mammas: her blonde pageboy hairstyle created a sort of halo around her face, and her curvy figure and bubbly presence made her one of those people who pulled you into her inner circle from her first hello.

I stammered as I explained my appearance to her. When I was done, Karin tossed back her head and laughed—not in a mocking way, but in a way that got me laughing at myself. In her lovely Danish accent—which reminded me of Irene Dunne in the 1948 movie *I Remember Mamma*—she told me not to worry, but to go home, change, and come back. She exuded motherly support.

No reprimand?

I exhaled.

No punishment for being less than perfect?
Karin said to go home and come back. Come back!
You looked a mess.
I did, and it was okay, I thought, laughing to myself.

PAPÀ COULDN'T HAVE BEEN MORE proud of me. His daughter was a writer working for a newspaper. I felt pretty pleased with myself, too. I'd race home every Monday through Friday and share the highlights of my day with him. He'd sit for hours, his eyes wide and full of love, listening, laughing, and praising. No wonder he assumed I was more than happy exactly where I was—which is what led him to do what he did.

On one of those days, I came home to find a scribbled message from Papà on a notepad left near the kitchen phone. It read: *"Paola—Oopah call for job."*

Oopah? I thought to myself. Did he mean Oprah?

When I asked Papà for details, he couldn't confirm anything other than that the person calling had been a very nice lady with a name that sounded something like "Oopah"; he said that I wasn't to worry, since he'd told her that I was no longer looking for a job and already had a big job I loved as a writer at a newspaper.

You have got to be kidding! I screamed within. But the glow of pride on his face when he told me prohibited me from telling him how much I wish he hadn't done what he had.

As much as it was true that I did love my new job at the newspaper, it also was true that I would have jumped in a heartbeat at the chance to interview to work for Oprah. Who in their right mind wouldn't?

I called Harpo Productions and explained that I thought Oprah had called me for a job. As I said the words, even I thought I sounded like a lunatic. I was told to leave my name and number and they would call back if, indeed, she had.

Needless to say, that never happened. Once again, whether Oprah really had or hadn't called me, my family seemed to always get in the way of my being able to live my own life.

IN TERMS OF LIFE AT THE NEWSPAPER, however, I took to it just as Dorothy took to landing in Oz. Everything exploded with color. From the people to the production plant to seeing one of my first copywriting pieces in print, it was all so new and exciting. Fear never came into play, only curiosity. I had found my yellow brick road and was on my way to finding where I belonged—the place I could finally feel was my home.

My role as a copywriter, helping to promote the newspaper, grew into writing feature stories about events and everyday Janes and Joes who had a story to tell. I also got to collaborate on the paper's special sections, working with teammates on cover concepts and writing the accompanying stories. I even graduated to having my own column, writing on any topic I wanted, and getting published in a tri-city area three times each week.

Before long, my cubicle, which I had adorned with inspirational quotes and printed schedules detailing every deadline I had to hit, felt more like home than my actual home. And my colleagues felt like family.

When Jimmy Stewart published his book of poems and held a book signing at Kroch's and Brentano's in Chicago's Water Tower Place on the famed Magnificent Mile, Karin let me go to interview him and do a story for our upcoming holiday gift guide. Standing in line with a press pass, about to talk to George Bailey himself, I felt as if I would faint.

What questions I asked? What answers he gave? I remember none of it, but do remember the feeling of kindness and warmth that he exuded.

Upon returning home, I sent Jimmy a thank-you note, gushing about having met my idol. I also gifted him with a brass belt buckle similar to the one Janet from ISU's Animal Ecology Department had worn; this one, however, depicted a horse that looked just like Pie, Jimmy's costar of twenty-two years. I never expected to get a hand-written note from Jimmy Stewart in response, but I did, and I couldn't have wished for a greater gift that Christmas. I felt as if I was in my own version of *It's A Wonderful Life*.

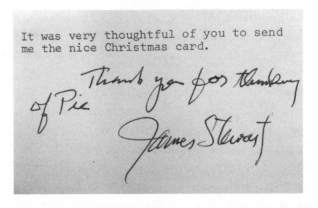

It was very thoughtful of you to send
me the nice Christmas card.

of Pic

Thank you for thinking of Pic

James Stewart

Well in advance of the holiday shopping season, the team of creatives I worked with was tasked with coming up with some sort of program to kick off the newspaper's gift guide series. We needed something to boost the newspaper's sales, and to motivate internal staff to get into the spirit of the season months before Christmas shopping would even begin. So I started dreaming up a silly idea to pitch to the sales team.

"We do a parody of *It's A Wonderful Life* but call it *'Twas The Night Before Deadline—The Musical!*"

I could see the faces of my dozen or so coworkers crinkling, their eyebrows furred and lips skewed, all of them trying to wrap their minds around what I was suggesting. I had started writing out a script, and I shared it to help them better understand my idea.

Jimmy, my favorite sales rep, looked like a gangster but had the heart of a jester. He immediately came to mind to play the lead of Clarence, the angel trying to get his wings and who had "the IQ of a rabbit but the faith of a child."

I explained further by saying our musical would follow a sales rep who, like George Bailey, had become discouraged by his lack of sales and the fact that the time to make his sales quota was running out. On the night before Christmas, he'd be visited by other characters, similar to *A Christmas Carol*'s ghosts of past, present, and future, who would inspire him with reasons to sell, show him what a wonderful life it is, and convince him that it could be made even *more* wonderful by hitting his goals and earning prizes.

Throughout the skit, we'd sing famous tunes with lyrics I'd revised: "We Need A Little Christmas" became "Roll out the Gift Guides"; the Bee Gee's "Staying Alive" became a song about "Getting Those Ads"; and the grand finale, "Gift Guide Time," was sung to the tune of *Jesus Christ, Superstar*'s theme song.

It was wacky, but they all bought into it, and we shined. I felt like a superstar. The Paddock Players, the name we had given ourselves, all pointed to me as the leader of our creative ensemble. Everyone at work—including my boss, Karin, and the owners of the newspaper, Margie, Bob, and Stu Paddock—gave our performance a standing ovation. And each one shook my hand and congratulated me.

Me!

Stuart Paddock, Sr., my favorite of the three siblings, held my hand in his after the show. He smiled, looking very much like Santa Claus with his white hair, rosy red cheeks, and rounded belly, and said, "You, young lady, are a rising star!"

I felt just as I had in Lee's writing class back at ISU.

AT HOME, I WAS DETERMINED to entertain and bring joy, too, just like my papà.

Papà loved to perform. He'd spend hours sitting with his mandolin, playing self-taught tunes like "Love Theme" from *The Godfather*. He attempted to teach me to play the instrument, patiently showing me where to put my fingers to play "Tu Scendi Dalle Stelle," the one tune I did manage to learn. Or he'd listen to his operas and conduct imaginary orchestras, making me laugh while he pretended to direct his favorite tenor, Luciano Pavarotti, in singing Puccini's aria "Nessun Dorma." Rising to his feet, tears in his eyes, his mouth wide open, he'd sing the final words—"*Vincerò, Vincerà, Vincerò*"—with gusto.

Most of the time, Mamma slept. Her rage had calmed down. For now, or so it seemed, the drug cocktail she had been prescribed was keeping her somewhat more functional than less, more even-keeled than out of control.

Viny, on the other hand, was still rebelling against any restrictions on her freedom. Now twenty-two years old, she had gotten it into her head that she could be out on her own. When some scam of a sales venture offered her a seasonal position touring the United States and going door-to-door to sell who knows what, she fought to join. It was just the latest of her tantrums, and of Papà forbidding her from following through on the crazy ideas she wanted to pursue.

The two battled often.

The screaming between them would only come to a cease-fire when Papà stopped to catch his breath, one hand held over his heart, and declared to her, "*Un giorno mi farai morire di un attacco di cuore!*"

Despite my papà's angry words, telling Viny she would one day cause him to die from a heart attack, the two always made up. Viny would apologize for not knowing what had gotten into her, and Papà would sigh, not knowing what to do with her.

EMOTIONS RAN HIGH IN OUR HOME. Maybe it was just a cultural thing. Maybe it was something more. I tried to keep my own spirits in check and focus on my job. I pretended to the outside world that I went home to normal, that *I* was normal.

Nothing to see here.

I was still winning the war, keeping crazy at bay.

ON NOVEMBER 9 OF THAT YEAR, another war—or the end of one—was all over the news. On that Thursday night, I sat on the couch, curled up with my papà in the living room, and witnessed the fall of the Berlin Wall.

People of all ages, bundled up in their winter jackets, stood atop a concrete wall tagged from top to bottom with colorful graffiti. What those words said, I did not know. But the smiles and chatter of the men and women pulling one another up to cross over or to stand side by side on the wall's top ledge; the sight of pickaxes, chisels, and sledgehammers breaking off chunks and pieces of concrete; the eruption of cheers once they broke through the wall to the other side—all of it moved Papà to tears. East and West Berlin were separated no more.

"Non avrei mai pensato di vedere . . ."

Papà wept at what he said he'd never thought he would see.

I stared at his weathered face, the glow of the TV screen adding a shimmer to the tears that pooled in the crevices of his wrinkles. His eyes were fixated on the scenes unfolding before us. I knew very little about communism and next to nothing of the fascist world both Papà and Mamma had grown up in: Hitler and Mussolini had ruled for much of their time living in Sicily. So, too, had the Mafia.

"Meglio partire che morire." One reason Papà always gave as to why he chose to leave his beloved home. "Better to leave than to die."

PAPÀ NEVER DWELLED ON WHAT HAD been or on what he wished could be. He rejoiced in simply being. He celebrated every moment there was to celebrate. While he'd always felt comfortable expressing his emotions, however, the older he got, the more weepy he seemed to be.

And when we watched for the millionth time our favorite Christmas movie, *It's A Wonderful Life*, that year, for some reason those tinkling angel bells that usually comforted me, reminding me of Clarence finally getting his wings, didn't. Instead, they gave rise within me the feeling that something was wrong.

"Papà, che c'è?"

Now it was my turn to ask him what was wrong. A part of me expected him to answer as I always did, with a simple "nothing"; however, after he searched my face for an uncomfortably long few moments—for what, exactly, I don't know—he finally exhaled, leaned closer to me, and whispered one word: "Cancer."

FOR MONTHS, I LEARNED, ROSARIO had been escorting Papà to an oncologist for treatment of bladder cancer. And for those same months, I'd known nothing, other than the fact that Papà seemed to have to urinate more often than usual.

Why weren't you paying attention?

All you thought about was you: superstar.

No way can you leave him now.

Papà would need me now more than ever before. So, too, would Viny.

My little sister shrugged at the news. "He'll be fine," she said, a wry smile on her lips.

Her cavalier attitude suggested she didn't care. But I knew that wasn't it. She just didn't want to think of any other possibility. Nor did I. Papà was indestructible, a man of superhuman strength.

What if he's not?

I refused to hear the whispers of doubt and fear. And playing my part as big sister, I attempted to distract Viny from all of her crazy thoughts by taking her to see Disney's latest animated release, *The Little Mermaid.*

"It's my life, Pauley," Viny argued with me as we sat in the movie theater, waiting for the film to start. "I'm old enough. I should be able to do what I want."

She was right: it was her life, she was old enough, and she should be able to do what she wanted. I knew how she felt, feeling much the same way. But in Viny's case, her age didn't match her knowledge or maturity. She was still at a pre-teen level in terms of being able to reason and fend for herself. Everyone she met was someone she immediately trusted. Admirable, yes, but it often put her at risk. Meanwhile, basic living skills—cooking, doing laundry, washing her own hair—were too much for her. Even when getting popcorn and soda at the concession stand for the movie, she had no idea how much money she needed or how much change back to expect. She was easy prey for others who were out to take advantage of her. And more often than not, they did. How would she ever survive on her own?

It was a thought that plagued me as much as if not more so than Mamma and her mental illness. It was why I'd pushed so hard to get Viny enrolled in special services. But Rosario thought Viny's bad behavior was due to that Pioneer Center. He'd never thought putting her in the program was a good idea, and now he put the blame squarely on me for ever having initiated doing so.

But somewhere deep within me, I knew that if I didn't start her in something that gave her a chance at living independently now, I would be the one stuck caring for her down the road. And that couldn't happen. It was another "it" I feared.

The lights dimmed and the movie began to play. Sixteen-year-old Ariel wanted to live her own life, too, as a human out of the sea and on dry land. Her father, King Triton, forbade it, but Ariel went ahead and did what she wanted anyway.

As much as Ariel's story matched what Viny was living, I chuckled at the ironies, parallels and disconnects in my own life: losing your voice, bartering for what you wanted, having a papà who would give his own life for yours. While I had treated Viny to *The Little Mermaid* in the hopes of quieting her rebellion, the opposite proved true for her. The story also served to rekindle my own dreams—I wanted to be somewhere else and someone other than me.

Life's not a fairy tale.
You're stuck where you are.

CHAPTER FOURTEEN: **COUNTDOWN**

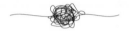

"GUARDA, PAPÀ!" I SHOUTED excitedly, plopping down on the couch next to where he sat gently rocking in his recliner. The Saturday *Daily Herald* had just been delivered, and right there on the front page of the newspaper was a photograph of an eleven-year-old girl and an article about how she was living her life to the fullest despite having to manage an ostomy bag.

I spread open the page and laid it out over his lap, making sure not to disturb the bulge of his own ostomy bag—lest it leak, again. Bladder cancer had threatened to rob Papà of his life. The doctors had promised they'd save him with a simple surgery to remove it. In its place, they'd leave him with a hole on his right side under his belly, allowing his urine to leave his body and be collected into a pouch that affixed to his skin. All he had to do was empty it several times each day.

Once again, the doctors hadn't known best. They'd assumed that because Papà was seventy-three years old, he lived a sedentary life. Rosario had argued with the doctors to enclose the ostomy bag inside rather than affixing it outside the body; unfortunately, that wasn't what had happened. And the pouch that was supposed to stay put never seemed to. Every time Papà bent over in his garden or went for a bike ride, his ostomy bag would leak. He raged against it, his face turning red, tears filling his eyes. As a result, he spent less and less time outdoors. He resigned from his job at Dominick's grocery store. And even on warm, sunny days, with his beloved garden beckoning, he frequently chose to stay indoors.

"*No, Paola.*" He looked up from the smiling child in the article, his own face a reflection of despair. "*La bimba non sa ancora cosa significha avera questa borsa cazza, perche non ha ancora vissuto esperienza della vita.*"

As I looked into my papà's sad eyes, a scene from *It's A Wonderful Life* popped into my head: God tells the angel Clarence that a man on Earth needs their help. Clarence asks if the man is sick and God replies, "No, worse. He's discouraged." Papà's insight about the eleven-year-old in the newspaper article not knowing what it really meant to have a shitty ostomy bag because she hadn't had enough life experience yet shattered my heart. While the cancer may not have taken Papà's life, the surgeons had.

BY THE TIME PALM SUNDAY ROLLED around that year, Papà had resigned himself to living his life with that ostomy bag. He sat in his recliner, transforming the green reeds he had brought home from Mass into the shapes he knew and we loved best. He handed me my pinecone basket to replace the previous year's, which had somewhat disintegrated over time while hanging on the mirror in my room.

As I swapped them out, I studied my reflection. My aunt Rose, the one who had taken Viny in while I was away at ISU, had always said I was like the moon—my face so big and round and shining.

She's trying not to say what you really are: fat.
You need to get a life.

It was true. I was obese, at least 100 pounds overweight. At home, when Viny and Papà argued, I ate. Papà's melancholy broke my heart, which I comforted with food and booze. And Mamma's mood swings had me stuffing my face even more. I did have my job at the newspaper, but I wanted more. My frustrations spilled over into the office, and I felt as if even there, my shine had faded. Lifeless eyes looked back at me from my mirror. I needed to get out of this house and into a place of my own.

Always be nasty.

FOR BOTH MOTHER'S DAY AND Father's Day that year, I refused to be the sibling who ordered the cakes, made the reservations at restaurants, and selected possibilities for giving a joint gift to our parents on their respective days. I wanted out. Papà had hinted that he wanted an electric drill. I pretended not to understand him. Instead of shopping for his gift that year, I shopped for myself, touring apartments I might be able to afford on my own. And I kept my plans a secret.

For weeks, I had been keeping another secret from Papà, one with Rosario's help. The *Daily Herald*'s Father's Day Gift Guide needed a model we could dress up and pose for the accompanying feature story I was writing on crazy Father's Day gifts. I had pitched the idea to the team, not disclosing my expertise on the topic of crazy in a mental-illness-of-Mamma or madness-at-home kind of way; rather, I focused on the silly, foolish, ridiculous, looney-toon kind of meaning normally associated with the word and the holiday.

The irony made me laugh at myself.

So did the resulting cover photo.

Rosario fit the newspaper's criteria for gender and age range, and he looked as if he actually could be someone's father. Most importantly, he agreed to model for free. We dressed him up in some of Papà's favorite articles of clothing, including his signature grey tweed flat cap.

The special section featuring Rosario on its cover, dressed like Papà and with a disappointed look on his face and, holding up an ugly necktie as his gift, published on June 13, just four days prior to Father's Day. Rosario's actual expression upon seeing himself in the newspaper also registered disappointment; he clearly regretted saying yes to modeling. Papà, on the other hand, beamed at the sight of his only son featured on the newspaper's front page along-side the story that his *Paolamia* had written.

Before we even sat down to celebrate with cake, Papà went out to buy up all the copies at the local White Hen convenience store. He drove all over town, proudly showing off to the people at Dominick's and the guys at the gas station where he pumped gas and anyone anywhere else who happened to be someplace where the paper with his son's face was sold, telling them that *this* was *his* boy.

Surrounded by his family, celebrating his day, Papà glowed. A part of me wanted to stay forever. I would miss him the most when I moved out. And when I did, he would be left on his own to care for Mamma and Viny.

Not your problem.

He left his family in Sicily. He'll understand.

"Che pensi, Paolamia?"

He always wanted to know what I was thinking.

"Niente, Papà."

Nothing to see here.

ON THE THURSDAY AFTER FATHER'S Day, I woke up, showered, and made my way into the kitchen for breakfast. As usual, Papà was up, already pouring me a cup of coffee and asking me what I wanted to eat. I kissed him good morning and sat down at our kitchen table. My back was to him, but I could hear the cracking of eggs and the sizzling of butter as he plopped them into the frying pan.

Casually, he said, *"Sai, ho sognato la nonna ieri sera."*

I sipped my coffee, not thinking much of Papà's telling me he had dreamt about his mother, my grandmother, that night. Papà had told me many times before how much I reminded him of *la nonna*, saying our similarities weren't just in our size but our per-sonalities. I, he said, did just as *la nonna* had: I pointed out things others missed or simply couldn't see. Not visions or spirits, like Mamma, but clouds that looked like thundering horses, or baby bunnies born and hiding in the backyard, or tiny violets that had no business growing in concrete. Whenever he spoke of his own mamma, tears came to Papà's eyes. He loved her so.

"*Mi ha baciato sulle labra*," he continued.

I felt the hairs on my arms tingle. It took me a minute to respond, and did so only after swallowing more of my coffee.

"Grandma kissed you on the lips?" I thought of what he had said, trying to keep my cool, despite knowing full well what Sicilian folklore foretold: dreaming of the person you loved most who had crossed over kissing you on the lips meant that in three days, you would be joining them.

Papà laughed. "*Tre giorni*," he said, running his index finger across his throat and making a guttural, slicing sound while hanging his tongue out in mock murder.

"*Ma tu non ci credi in quello, vero?*" Trying to keep my words free from the unexpected sense of fear that had just risen up within me, I scoffed, asking to make sure he didn't believe in such nonsense.

"*No!*" He chuckled and whispered, "*Non dirlo alla mamma.*"

I agreed I wouldn't tell Mamma. She believed in all sorts of superstitions, and this would send her into a panic. Having grown up in the little town of Nicosia, known for its irrational beliefs and white magic makers, Mamma surely would believe the dream to be a sign, a very bad sign . . . and the rest of us would suffer for it.

THE FOLLOWING NIGHT, FRIDAY, I went out with friends and returned home quite late. After I entered the house, closed the door behind me, and climbed the stairs, I found Papà sitting up and waiting for me. The room was dark, apart from the glow of the TV.

I dropped my bags at the top of the landing, walked over to where Papà sat on his recliner, and plopped myself down on the couch to his right.

"*Ti sei divertita?*" Papa's glasses reflected ghostly images from the scenes playing out on the screen as he rocked his recliner forward to mute the sound.

I nodded, letting him know I did have a good time.

Moments later, the portable phone that sat in its cradle in front of us on the marble coffee table began to chirp and beep. Its screeching seemed as if it was trying to make a connection all on its own, with a dial tone and the bizarre transmission of pieces of conversations we couldn't quite make out.

Papà and I exchanged glances and laughed at the otherworldly sounds.

"*Sono gli spiriti*," he joked.

I nervously laughed at his comment about the sounds being from spirits. It reminded me of our earlier conversation.

"*Hai paura di morire?*" I didn't intend to ask him if he was afraid to die. The question just fell out of my mouth.

Without hesitation, Papà responded, almost as if he had been asking and answering the same of himself for hours: "*Affatto. Ho la mia famiglia. Ho fatto tanto. Ho vissuto una vita meravigliosa. Sono pronto a vedere cos'altro c'è da vedere.*"

I sat in silence, letting his words sink in. On the one hand, I was happy that he wasn't at all afraid to die, that he felt he had done so much, had his family, and had lived a wonderful life. On the other hand, him saying he was ready to see what else there was to see unnerved me.

Papà turned to me, his face full of light, his expression almost excited. "*Vuoi che torno e ti dico com'è?*"

I half laughed, half cringed. "Okay," I said and shrugged, feeling uneasy at him asking me if I wanted him to come back and tell me what the afterlife was like. "*Ma, non mi fare spaventare.*"

Just as I asked him to not scare me upon his return from the dead, whatever conversations were transmitting through the phone suddenly ceased. Dead silence. Papà widened his eyes, raised his eyebrows, and put his finger to his lips, shushing me.

I laughed, shaking my head. Then I rose, kissed him on his cheek, and bid him good night.

THE NEXT MORNING, SATURDAY, I wasn't feeling all that great. I fought through the chills and my lower backache so I could attend a screenwriting seminar in Chicago for which I had registered months earlier. In slow motion, I showered, dressed, and made my way outside to the garden to kiss Papà good-bye. As I approached, Papà stood in front of his precious grape vine, his back to me. In spite of my body's growing pain, I chuckled, reminded that this was the year Papà would get to pick his beloved grapes and finally taste the fruits, literally, of his years of labor. Those grapes reignited his passion to spend time in his garden. Where else would he be this morning but outside, admiring his babies and envisioning *il vino dolce* that they were destined to become?

He turned to face me, and the look on his face was one of such profound sorrow that I skipped a step and almost came to a complete stop. My eyes shifted from his to what was no longer obscured from my view: His ancient vine, which just yesterday had been bursting with plump, ripe, golden fruits, was now barren. The grapes had disappeared, and it was clear that Papà had not been the one to pick them.

"*Disgraziate!*" Papà spewed, calling the thieves responsible wretched.

"Oh, Papà!" I didn't know what I could possibly say that would matter. I shrugged ever so slightly and then hugged and kissed him, telling him I needed to get going or I'd be late.

"*Vai, vai, Paolamia,*" he waved me off. "*Diverteti. Gente miserabili! Aspetiamo un altro anno, eh?*"

Leaving him, even with him telling me to go and have fun, didn't feel right, but I went anyway. What miserable people would do such a thing? At least Papà was moving on already, saying we'd just have to wait one more year.

BY MID-MORNING AT THE conference, I could barely sit or stand or pay attention. As much as I tried to hang on, I couldn't.

I went home and immediately climbed into bed.

SUNDAY MORNING, I SLEPT IN. Papà came into my room to check on me. He made funny faces and promised to make my favorite Pasta Fina Fina, Italian chicken soup. *That*, he said, would fix me right up. I gave him a weary smile, and he left my room to head outside.

From my window, I could hear Rosario and Papà laughing outside. I painfully turned my body to peek through the blinds. Rosario was showing off a brand-new car, a dark blue Ford Taurus. He had just bought it that morning, I could hear him saying. It was quite a scene: he and Papà walking around and around its exterior, admiring the shine, opening the doors, and Papà exaggerating his breathing, commenting on that new car smell. Rosario was twenty-eight now, and Papà's pride and joy. He exuded it in his voice, his visage, his stance, and in how he looked at his son. Rosario oozed confidence and that thing that comes with knowing that the one person you love more than anyone else in this world not only loves you more but also approves of and celebrates everything about you.

Papà excitedly repeated the words "boo-tee-ful" and "*auguri*." From what I could hear, Rosario would be back soon to take Papà on a test drive. For now, he had come to borrow the lawn mower so he could cut the grass at his vacant lots out in Crystal Lake. It was Rosario's dream to build a home of his own design on that land: "The start of my empire," as he often said.

He departed, and I dozed off to sleep.

AROUND 11:00 A.M., MAMMA CAME into my bedroom, woke me, and calmly told me Papà didn't feel well. He wanted me to call an ambulance. I jumped out of bed, hurried to our kitchen phone, and called. Papà sat on his recliner; he whispered something to Mamma as she hovered over him, obscuring my vision. I heard her offering him a cup of tea.

"Yes, my father's still conscious," I responded to the 911 operator on the other end of the phone. "He's even talking."

I hung up the receiver and started back to my bedroom, calling over my shoulder to my parents that an ambulance was on its way. I never bothered to look at Papà's face as I passed him by. No worry nor any concerns entered my mind. No feelings of fear whatsoever churned inside me. Even the voices were silent.

I had stepped out of my pajamas and was pulling on my pants and shirt when I heard a loud bang and a panicked-sounding Mamma calling out Papà's name, then mine. I raced out of my room and the few feet halfway down the hall to where Mamma stood. Her eyes were wide with fear and tears trickled from their corners. "*Subito, Paola!*" She pointed inside the bathroom.

There on the white-tiled floor, wedged into the less than two-foot space between the toilet and the bathtub, lying on his back, with a stream of vomit running down his chin, was my papà.

I had seen this before, on the night my uncle Joe died with these very same signs. Three words echoed in my head as my insides convulsed: *massive heart attack.*

Shaking my head, forcing myself to move, I barked orders to the only other person there. I wanted to call 911 again: "*Il telefono, Mamma!*"

You should have sounded more urgent!

Damning thoughts echoed within.

I, again, was the adult in charge. Mamma's sobs and her calling out Papà's name echoed throughout the house as she scurried to bring me the phone. I knelt at Papà's side and placed my mouth over his, struggling to control my gagging as I tried to ignore what I was tasting and focused on what I was doing: pretending.

I didn't want to believe it, but I already knew that Papà was gone. I was too late. Yes, I was trying to save him, but it was all just panic and, despite the motions, pretend. I kept at the CPR anyway, instinctively knowing that if I did not at least appear to be doing something, I would forever be looked at askance by the rest of the family, the question always written on their faces: "Why didn't you try to save him?"

Seconds later, as I pushed down again on Papà's chest, my hands overlapping one another, I felt a force physically push me away from him. I paused, dismissing it as my imagination, and tried to lean forward toward him again—but once more, something wasn't having it. It felt as if two hands were now on me, one on my chest and the other at my back, both gently but steadily pushing me and pulling me back. I sat on my haunches, almost expecting to see whatever it was that was present with me in that room, but there was nothing. Just Papà and me.

I stared at his ashen face. Something inside me whispered that he wasn't there in that body, not anymore. I breathed in, a calm sense of peace washing over me.

"*Paola*!" Mamma shouted.

I snapped to. Vomit continued to trail out of Papà's mouth, trickling down his chin and cheek. I reached up to the counter, grabbed a wash cloth that sat near the sink, and wet it, then used it to wipe away what I could. My hand brushed the side of his face, already so cold to my touch, further confirming for me that he was gone.

TWO YOUNG MALE PARAMEDICS, along with another older man who said he was the emergency medical technician arrived and entered the house. They asked Mamma and me to wait outside. Mamma started down the steps from the living room; I trailed behind. Turning my head back, I saw the two medics drag my papà by his feet out of the bathroom to the hallway, where they began working on him. The EMT grabbed me by the arm just as I was about to take the first step down the staircase.

"It doesn't look good," he whispered, staring intently into my eyes.

My head nodded in slow motion, and I heard myself calmly respond to him, "I know. He's already dead."

By the time I met up with Mamma outside in the driveway, several neighbors had gathered close to her. The ambulance's flashing lights danced from face to face, each one a different slant of shock and sadness. No one spoke but for faint whispers and escaped whimpers.

The EMT pushed open the front door's screen, as the paramedics carried Papà's 250-plus-pound body out on a stretcher. A gasp escaped us all as they nearly dropped him trying to maneuver down the front steps of the house.

As we watched, I heard the sounds of an engine revving toward us and then screeching to a stop against the curb. Caterina flung open her passenger door and nearly tumbled out. Her face registered disbelief, then a flash of rage, as she made her way to me.

"Why didn't you call the ambulance sooner?" she screamed at me, tears now starting to flow down her cheeks.

Her words were like a knife to my heart.

Why didn't you call the ambulance sooner?

You took your sweet time getting dressed.

"He's still talking"—why did you say that?

How could you have stopped doing CPR?

So many accusations from within already indicting me; hers, I did not need.

Lights flashing, sirens still screaming, well aware of our many witnesses, I waited until my sister was so close to me I could feel her heat, and then I said in the most quiet yet deadly sounding, low-pitched voice I could muster, "You were a bitch when Papà was alive, and you're still a bitch now; if you say one more word, I'll punch you in your fucking face."

I'm not sure why I chose those words. I doubt I would have punched her, even if she deserved it. I was able to conjure up the most vicious of words to wound—words that actually succeeded in silencing both my sister and my own choir of critics.

Was this how normal people behaved, reacting to this kind of crisis? Did everyone talk to family this way? Just a few days ago, we'd all been together for Father's Day, so happy. How had we gotten here?

Mamma rode in the ambulance with Papà; they said they would be taking him to Sherman Hospital in Elgin, a twenty-minute ride away. My sister's husband volunteered to drive to Crystal Lake to find Rosario and give him the news.

Caterina and I left together in my car to get Viny from her job near the local mall. My mind calculated distance and time:

fifteen minutes to arrive at the restaurant where Viny worked; more minutes for us to run inside, explain the situation to Viny and her bosses, collect our little sister, and get back to the car; then another fifteen minutes to drive to the hospital emergency room. That would be close to an hour that Papà would already have been dead by the time we got there.

I don't recall the drive. I don't remember if my sisters and I said anything to one another. I don't remember parking the car when we arrived at the hospital. Nor do I know where my sisters went or why I was the only one the medical staff allowed into the little room where they had put Mamma to wait for news about Papà.

What I do remember is sitting with Mamma in what had to be two of the most uncomfortable plastic chairs ever. Maybe it was the pain I still felt in my back. But Mamma squirmed too, her legs shaking underneath the folding table that stretched out in front of us. She turned toward me and raised her once-beautiful hands—now gnarled from her growing arthritis—with a look of hope on her face, even as her eyes welled up with tears, and asked me if I thought Papà would be alright.

I knew he wouldn't be, but I couldn't bring myself to immediately respond.

Just then, the door to the room opened wide.

I was grateful for the intrusion.

A man dressed in dark blue surgical scrubs darted in. He pulled out one of the other chairs, sat down to the left of Mamma, and matter-of-factly started speaking. I watched his lips moving; the rest of his face was a blur. The words I heard somehow seemed out of sync with the movements of his mouth.

"We did everything we could," he began. "Your husband, however, expired."

Mamma threw up her hands, tossed back her head, and exclaimed, "Oh! Tanka God."

I stifled a very inappropriate laugh at the sound of Mamma thanking God and gave a very dirty look to the messenger.

Who the hell uses the word "expired"?

He wasn't a carton of milk that went bad.

"My mother doesn't understand English very well," I found myself calmly explaining to the faceless man, resisting the urge to chastise him for his insensitivity and poor use of words. Then I turned to look at Mamma in the eye and softly said, "*Mamma, Papà è morto.*"

Saying the words out loud to Mamma—Papà is dead—numbed me. Far off in the distance, I could hear Mamma's wailing, and her repeated plea of "No" and question of "Why?" My eyes blurred over with tears, morphing both her and the doctor into one giant smudge.

WHAT SEEMED LIKE MINUTES LATER, we all were marched down a long corridor. On either side of us, behind soundproof glass, medical teams were gathered. I could see all of them talking and laughing with one another as if nothing important had just happened. To them, everything was normal. I wanted to storm into those rooms and scream at them. The one person who made things as normal as they could be for us was now gone. How could they be laughing?

At the end of our death march, we were escorted into a room where Papà was laid out on a stainless steel table with wheels. Flashes of Charlie ran through my mind. I would never let anyone carve up my papà.

He was covered up to his neck with a light blue sheet. His tanned complexion had turned the color of putty. His features were hardened. His face didn't look like him. He was there in front of us, and yet, he clearly wasn't.

I don't know what we all said or how long it was before we left Papà all alone in that room. I imagine we each said our good-byes before heading home without him.

Mamma and my two sisters rode in one car with my brother-in-law driving. Rosario and I walked toward my car. He put his arm around me and drew me in. He asked me if I felt up to driving. I didn't. He did.

As we drove down Route 25, we passed the little cemetery

Papà had said he wanted to be buried in. As I pointed it out to Rosario, I caught myself waving. My brother laughed, then pointed upward to two billowy clouds that hung low in the sky. Each one looked as if it had taken on a human form. One of them almost looked like the Pillsbury Dough Boy, the little Poppin' Fresh figure that wore a baker's cap. Papà would always mimic his giggle and poke at his own belly whenever the mascot appeared in some TV commercial. The other cloud was much bigger, and it looked as if the two were holding hands.

"Look," Rosario said, trying not to choke up. "It's like the big one's helping the little one, pulling him along."

I nodded, losing the battle not to cry myself. I thought of the stories Papà told of when he was a little boy in Sicily. He said he would lie on his back in the grass and watch the clouds float on by. He would pretend he could jump high enough to hop onto a cloud, and he dreamed of riding it across the ocean all the way to America.

ONCE HOME, WE ALL GATHERED in the living room. Mamma and I sat on the couch. Viny sat on the broken chair at the dining room table, across from our brother-in-law; they were both absolutely silent. Rosario and Caterina stood, sometimes pacing. Papà's empty chair, his rocker recliner, sat motionless.

My two older siblings began their questioning, demanding answers to: What happened? How could this have happened? Didn't you see any signs? When did he start feeling sick? Why didn't you call then? When did he ask for an ambulance? How long did it take for the paramedics to get here? Did you do CPR? For how long?

I felt as if I was standing trial. The questions were understandable, but the accusatory tone was only feeding my own voices, which had already decided I was guilty on all counts. I answered truthfully, except I didn't dare tell them that I had stopped CPR soon after starting. They wouldn't have understood. I'm not quite sure I understood yet either.

"If I had been here, I would have cracked his chest open," Rosario declared in a Monday morning quarterbacking kind of way that made me feel like shit.

Viny soon disappeared from the room—silently slinking off to her bedroom and locking her door behind her. She, for sure, would be taking it hard. She battled with Papà so often.

But no one could have predicted this. Even Papà saying that Viny would give him a heart attack . . . it was all just talk. Not one of us had seen any signs that this was a possibility of coming true. At least not that I knew of.

"Meglio dire chissà che chi avrebbe potuto sapere."

How many times did Papà tell us, "Better to say 'who knows?' instead of 'who could have known?'"

You should have known.

The doorbell rang, interrupting the war raging in my own head. I needed to excuse myself from the impromptu inquisitions both outside and in, so I jumped up to answer whoever was at the front door. I ran down the stairs and pulled open our front door, which felt heavier than usual.

Karen, our neighbor from across the street and a few doors down who had befriended Papà, stood just outside. She and Papà shared a love for gardening. The two often exchanged vegetables and tips on how best to grow them. Her reddish hair and greenish eyes made me think she was Irish. Not that it mattered. Her eyes glistened as she struggled to say what she had come to say: "Is it okay if I pull some weeds out of your dad's garden?"

I stared at her for a moment. It was such an odd request. I thought I had misunderstood, but she repeated it again.

"I am so sorry," she added. "Your dad: I just loved him. We all loved him. Is it okay? The weeds? It'd be my way to honor your dad."

I nodded. Thanked her. She had always been Papà's favorite neighbor.

After shutting the door, I wondered for a split second how all the neighbors would survive without the annual summertime sharing of vegetables from my papà's garden. Then it dawned on me: How would his garden survive? How would I possibly keep it up?

THAT NIGHT, AS I LAY IN my bed, I tried to rewind the clock. Hours before he died. Days before. Weeks before. What was normal then hadn't really been normal. But what did that mean now? How much less than not normal could we be? Before all of this, I had been planning to move out. I needed to be on my own. But with him gone, how could I?

You can't.

You're stuck here.

I committed to staying just one year more, until I could be sure Mamma and Viny would be okay on their own. I would do it for Papà.

THE NEXT MORNING, I WOKE UP and headed into the kitchen. For a moment, I expected to see Papà pouring me my cup of coffee, and then I remembered what had happened. Picking up the phone's receiver, I dialed my boss' office number and left a message that I wouldn't be in because—I choked up on the words—my papà had died. I couldn't offer up much more.

Hanging up, swallowing back tears, I turned to face the empty kitchen. It was then that I saw it. There on the refrigerator door, my Papà had taped a note he had written on the back of one of the Father's Day cards he had received one week ago.

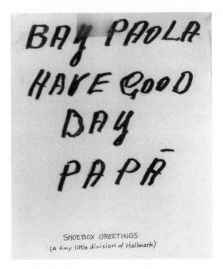

SHOEBOX GREETINGS
(A tiny little division of Hallmark)

CHAPTER FIFTEEN: **CAREGIVER**

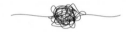

MADNESS HAD MADE ITSELF A member of our family. It had pulled up a chair at the dining room table one day long ago, bringing chaos as its dish to pass, and stayed to feast for nearly two decades. I expected it now, had almost gotten to the point of welcoming it. Crazy had become more comfortable than calm. It was normal—whereas quiet caused panic and the pins and needles of waiting for that other shoe to drop. Maybe that shoe would be a steel-toed leather boot capable of delivering a painful kick in the kidney, or maybe a sleek and spikey stiletto that could drive itself straight through the heart; whatever form it would take, I knew it would come, so I had to be ready for it.

What I failed to consider, however, was that the other shoe dropping would be in the form of Papà. His sudden death was more than a surprise; it was the fuzzy slipper that lulled me into slipping it on and snuggling into it, unaware of the venomous scorpion hiding inside. Papà had been the security blanket I always assumed would be with me. I had never really considered the possibility of him not. Nor had I thought of what I would do if he was taken from me.

Funeral arrangements need to be made.
Calls have to be placed to let others know.
Robotically, I made a list and set off to execute it.

BY THE FOLLOWING THURSDAY, I was sitting on a folding chair on the manicured lawn of the little cemetery across the street from the grocery store where Papà and I had shopped together. DOMINICK'S: the sign, with its bold, red letters and the red and green squiggles that went off to its sides seemed to wave at me. I had never looked at the storefront from that vantage point before.

I had never seen a grave up close before either. Severed roots poked through the earth where the hole had been dug. The closed bronze casket seemed to hover and shimmer in the sunlight. I thought of my papà inside, resting on the ivory velvet.

The funeral director said the concrete vault would make sure water wouldn't get in. Rosario's hand shook and his face grew white as he signed the paperwork allowing for Papà's blood to be replaced with embalming fluid.

Kissing Papà good-bye before they closed the casket, I noted how cold and gray he had become. He didn't look anything like himself. The life force he'd had inside before was for sure no longer. He was now just a hard, cold lump of clay. I wondered where the spark, the light, the soul that made Papà who he was had gone. Had it just disappeared forever? Was that it? It couldn't be.

Please don't let it be.

"Don't worry, sweetie. Soon you won't even remember what your dad looked like." The words someone had said while paying her respects echoed in my head.

Did she mean to be funny, like that Mary Tyler Moore episode? What a stupid thing to say.

I shut my eyes, committing every detail of Papà's face to memory.

I don't remember where Mamma or my siblings sat at the gravesite. Others showed up, but I couldn't say who. Someone shook my hand, saying that they hadn't even known Papà but had heard so much about him from the other neighbors that they wanted to pay their respects. People asked if he had been sick. I answered over and over that he wasn't. They were surprised to learn he was seventy-three years old. "He seemed so much younger." I heard that line over and over, too.

So many questions and comments; I nodded and smiled and made sure everyone else felt heard and cared for. In truth, I wished everyone would just disappear so I could fall apart.

MY WISH CAME TRUE.

Almost immediately, I found myself alone and forced to be in charge.

Rosario let go of anything he'd once thought mattered. The new car he had just bought was returned to the dealer. The properties he owned, the start of his empire, were sold. School and his ambitions of being an architect all died the day our papà did.

My two sisters retreated into their own respective worlds, as did Mamma. We all broke apart. But as the only one in the house who could even drive, someone had to pick up the slack. I reluctantly volunteered.

Days into living life without Papà, I did my best to become him: Mamma needed to be chauffeured to her doctor's appointments. Social security and social services for both her and Viny needed to be applied for. Household bills needed to be paid (the funeral had added $8,000 to the tab). Groceries had to be bought. The lawn had to be mowed. And Papà's once-thriving garden needed to be tended. Weeds were choking the life out of it, and I couldn't figure out how to keep it from dying either.

I never meant to abandon Papà's garden, just as I was sure Papà never meant to abandon me. He had said he'd come back to tell me how life on the other side was, but he hadn't yet delivered on his promise. Mamma said he had appeared to her, laughing and telling her that he was having a great time and had met Lucille Ball.

I wondered why he didn't share that with me.

I tried to immerse myself in my work at the newspaper, but not much of anything gave me any kind of joy anymore. I silently simmered with rage.

It's not fair.
Why him?
Why not Mamma?
Why me?

I cursed my fate, being left at home alone to not only resume my caregiver role as *la piccola mamma* but also to take on Papà's responsibilities. At work, watching coworkers excel, win praise, have fun with their friends, and live their own lives gave rise to envy within me. And if, even for a moment, I felt the tiniest glimmer of excitement or hope or happiness, guilt tortured me.

Don't you realize who's no longer around?
You should have tried harder to save him.
How can you be happy?
Mamma and Viny have nobody else.
You are stuck here.

On the outside, I projected as normal an image as I could muster—smiling, nodding, and participating in editorial meetings that no longer mattered to me. I pretended they did. I went through the motions as if my life had possibilities, despite having come to realize it didn't. On the inside, I could not escape the whispers that grew louder.

Would anyone care if you weren't around?
You could go be with Papà.
Keep it together.
You can't fall apart.

I feared my thoughts. They no longer seemed to be on this side of normal. And I no longer seemed able to control them.

I prayed, just in case anybody, including Papà, was listening: *Please don't let me be like Mamma.*

I could not share my feelings, let alone the life I went home to, with anyone. Our Sicilian family's unspoken code still ruled: What happened in the family, stayed in the family, a la *la cosa nostra*. I was committed now to live a life of obligation and servitude.

Money to keep up the house, help care for Mamma and Viny, and pay off my own debts never seemed to add up. Yet I couldn't stop spending. Every new project at work pushed me to ask for more money—or, if not that, at least more credit in the way of bylines and titles. My rising star was starting to fall. I fought with others, even coworkers I considered friends. And as everyone around me seemed to shine, my own light began to dim.

A few weeks into life without Papà, my boss Karin had had enough; she hauled me into her office one day and said loudly, "Paolina, I don't know what's gotten into you, but it's been ever since your father died!"

She was right. A cancer was growing; darkness was consuming my heart and soul. No matter how much I stuffed myself with pasta, bread, sweets, and alcohol, I couldn't ease the pain.

Friends tried to console me. Donna, for one, came over to coax me out for a ride one day, seemingly determined to drag me back among the living. As I sat inside the garage, its door wide open, I watched her drive up in her brand-new red convertible. She pushed open her car door, stepped out of it, and tentatively approached me while I continued to paint the wooden cross I had made out of two-by-fours.

"Hey, bud," she said. "Whatcha doin'?"

I stayed focused on my project. The hammered-in nails weren't as straight as I had hoped they'd be, so I filled in gaps with a second coat of white paint. "Temporary grave marker," I could barely be bothered to respond. The thought of Papà under the ground, with no sign of him being there, further made me feel as if he already was forgotten. I thought maybe that was why he had forgotten me.

Donna managed to get me to take a break from my amateur woodworking. Patrick Swayze, whom we had both lusted after ever since seeing him years before playing Johnny in *Dirty Dancing*, was starring in a movie that had just come out called *Ghost*. We took in a show. Sitting in the theater, watching Swayze's character Sam unexpectedly die and then try to communicate with the love he'd left behind, immediately flooded me with tears. Was Papà trying to find a way to talk to me? Had he just not figured out how yet?

When Whoopi Goldberg's character Oda Mae started hearing voices, my sobs turned into an uncontrollable laugh.

Get a grip! You're acting crazy.

Were my voices normal? Or like Mamma's?

Maybe they were like Oda Mae's?

I tried to swallow back my emotions, grateful to be sitting in a darkened theater.

My hand, resting in my lap, began to warm up. I kept my eyes on the movie screen. Slowly, it began to feel as if someone was holding my hand. The grip tightened, gently squeezing. Suddenly, I knew it was the comforting warmth and leathery touch of Papà's massive hand. The moment I looked down, however, the feeling left me.

Donna put her hand on my thigh and patted it. We exchanged glances in the dark—apology written all over her face, tears streaming down mine. I don't think either of us had realized what the movie was really about when we'd decided to go see it.

AFTER DONNA DROPPED ME OFF at home, I locked myself in my parents' bedroom. Mamma kept the family photo albums in her bottom dresser drawer. I pulled one out and stretched out onto Papà's side of the bed on my stomach to look at old photos of us. Almost immediately, an overpowering scent of the Musk cologne Papà always wore filled the room. I flipped over, fully expecting him to be standing there—and just like that, the smell completely vanished.

Papà? Is that you? Am I going crazy?

Mamma knocked on the door, startling me. "*Paola, che fai?*"

She wanted to know what I was doing. I did too.

I scrambled off the bed, tucked the photo album under my arm, and moved to unlock the door.

"*Niente, Mamma.*" I responded.

Nothing to see here.

She poked her head in and gave me an accusing look that was so familiar. Why the indictment was on her face at that particular moment, however, I didn't know.

Mamma acknowledged the photo album, nodding, as if she knew something I didn't. Her cryptic communications unnerved me. She gestured for me to sit on her bed. I did as she asked, fighting the urge to flee. I watched as she bent over to pull open the bottom drawer of her dresser and rummaged around, for what I had no clue. A few moments later, she extracted a few folders, each overstuffed with loose sheets of paper that I could see had writing all over them. She carried the files over and sat down alongside me.

Mamma leaned in and whispered in my ear. As I strained to hear what she had to say, I watched her eyes dart about, scanning the room, as if expecting someone else to be there.

"Dobbiamo stare zitti, o chissà ora che papà non è più qui cos'altro faranno."

I shut my eyes and inhaled, then exhaled with a loud sigh. "We have to stay silent," Mamma advised, because "who knows, with Papà now gone, what else they will do."

Mamma was clearly off her meds, talking nonsense again. *You should have been paying attention.*

"Ma . . ." I began as she handed me the files, but she cut me off by placing her finger to her lips, shushing me, and then rose without another word and slowly exited the room.

I made a mental note to call Rosario as soon as I could. No way was I going to get stuck taking care of crazy by myself. I could only imagine what she intended me to do with the pages she had just handed me. I pulled out a few to read.

The papers were Mamma's letters accusing doctors of experimenting on her, chastising Papà for his involvement, and threatening harm to him, to us, to herself. Each one I read escalated in rage. Scribbles in every direction filled the page, documenting delusions and speaking of phantoms who were "forcing her to speak" and act in certain ways.

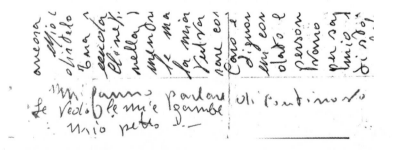

More careful cursives—moments of lucidity—painfully expressed Mamma's desperation. She wrote about Uncle Joe, hoping he could help her from beyond so that her children wouldn't lose their mother. She shared her love for her babies and her desire not to leave her husband who, she noted, was going through some bad times.

She ended crying out her plea: *"We were so happy, but unfortunately, the illness is destroying our home. God is with all!"*

Some letters were copied by hand, word-for-word, in triplicate. I shook my head at the utter confusion and pain. How sad for her and Papà. Just when she had started to stabilize a bit this past year, he, too, had been taken from her.

I pulled out more: love letters from Papà to Mamma.

"My Dear Maria, Our love is true, sincere and pure and there is no barrier that can crush it; what I say before God I swear, the more time passes and the more I want to love you. Your Antonino."

And not just from him to her but from her to him, reminiscing about their life together.

Mio amato Antonino;

Ricordo quando ci siamo visti per la prima volta, speravo che tu mi dicessi ti amo, più tardi si e realizzato il matrimonio e avere quattro figliuoli. Abbiamo fatto giornate e nottate ondolandoli per farli addormentare

"My beloved Antonino; I remember when we met for the first time. I was hoping you would tell me 'I love you'; later the marriage and having four children came true. We spent days and nights rocking them to sleep . . ."

At some point during my reading, I felt voyeuristic, as if spying on intimate interactions between two people who were my parents and yet were clearly strangers. I also felt a twinge of jealousy. I was supposed to be Papà's girl. This life of love between these two was something new for me to digest.

That's kind of sick.

Maybe Mamma was right to accuse you.

My own thoughts were jumbled.

Tucking their love letters away, I came upon the poems Papà had written and read to me back when I had come home from ISU for Christmas break. He had added to them, penning one I had not heard before about his love for Sicily. The poem began reminiscing about where he was born—its constant sunshine, the sparkle of the Mediterranean Sea, the return of springtime flowers, and how much he wanted to return home.

Oh! Sicilia mia Quanto sei bella!
nel tuo suolo le mie spoglie vorrei lasciare!

"Oh! My Sicily, how beautiful you are! In your soil, I would like to leave my remains."

Was this what Mamma had intended me to read? Were we supposed to ship Papà's body back to Custonaci, where he'd grown up?

When I turned the page over, I saw that Papà had also written a letter to the editor of the Italian newspaper *Fra Noi*.

se lo crede opportuno e ha dello spazio, sarei molto grato poter leggere il mio sonetto nel giornale fra noi.
Grazie anticipate,
Antonino Milana

"If you think it appropriate and have space, I would be most grateful to be able to read my sonnet in the *Fra Noi* newspaper."

Papà had never sent his letter. He'd probably been waiting for me to do what I had promised I would do: help him get published.

I had failed, had never even tried. Now, it was too late. He would never get to see his poem in the newspaper.

It's not too late.

You can still send it to Fra Noi.

I would. But it wouldn't be the same.

ONE MONTH TO THE DAY of Papà dying, I sat with friends in Chicago's Auditorium Theater, watching Andrew Lloyd Webber's *The Phantom of the Opera*. I bought the tickets months before, and as much as I didn't feel like it, I went.

"You promised. You promised." The girl in the musical, Christine, wept at her father's grave. He had promised to send his daughter the "Angel of Music" after his death, which he had not yet done.

Christine sang on stage about wishing her father was still there as I sobbed in my seat.

Later that night, home and all alone, I wrote to Papà, apologizing for my own broken promises. I told him that although he was gone, I would send his poems to the newspaper, and maybe he could see them published from wherever he was now. I also asked him to keep his promise:

She (Christine Baca) goes to her Father's grave & keeps saying "you promised" over & over.

It made me think of you — why don't you come to me & tell me everything O.K. I know you sent the scent but

I NEED TO HEAR THE WORDS.

I visited Papà's grave after work, as had become my habit. The morgue-like mood at home without him there was suffocating. Taking care of Mamma and Viny and pretending all was well required my almost daily fix of sitting in the grass beside him, the hump of dirt that covered him still not leveled. I brushed my hand over the clover that grew there in patches, telling him about my day and how much I missed him.

On this day I challenged him, though I didn't really put any force behind the words: "Papà, if you're here with me, let me find a four-leaf clover." My fingers plucked one tiny green plant at random. I blinked away tears, studied it . . . and counted its four leaves. "Thank you." I looked up to the sky, and carefully held my four-leaf clover in the palm of my hand, keeping it safe until I could press it in my journal back at home.

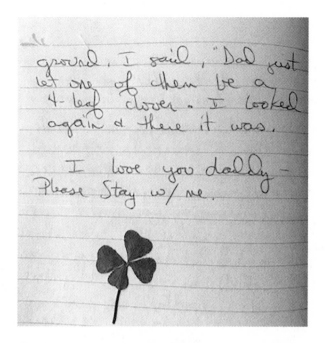

ground, I said, "Dad just
let one of them be a
4-leaf clover. I looked
again & there it was.

I love you daddy —
Please stay w/ me.

August 30, 1990. Two months had now passed since Papà's death. The connection he and I had shared seemed to have vanished right along with him. I no longer could feel him. He was no longer anywhere. It was as if he had never even existed.

I sobbed all alone in my car as I drove home from work. It had become part of my daily routine. I could barely see through my tears as I tried to make sure I didn't accidentally hit other cars, funneling my little white Escort into one of the lanes at the toll booth. I knew people in other cars could see me. Their looks of concern only made me angry. How could they carry on with their daily lives? Didn't they know my papà was dead? I wanted to shout the question out to them. Instead, I raised my voice to no one and pleaded, "Papà, where are you? Give me a sign, something, so I know you're still with me. Don't leave me, please."

No sooner had I whispered my prayer than a flashy compact car wedged its way in front of me. I slammed on my brakes and barely avoided bumping him. This—a near accident—was to be my answer? I felt in that moment what Jimmy Stewart's George

Bailey did when he asked, "Please, Father in Heaven, show me the way," only to get punched in the face by a man he did not know.

I swore at the sporty something that had cut me off as the driver tossed his coins into the tollbooth basket. It wasn't until he started to speed off that I noticed his license plate:

LUV DAD

Focusing, I reached out, gesturing with my hands. *Wait!* I was forced to brake behind the gate arm that lowered. Trying to keep my eyes on the car while tossing my coins into the basket, I lost him as he wove his way through traffic. What make or model was it? What color, even?

Had I really just seen what I thought I had? The sign I had asked for? The words I needed to see? The real answer to my prayer? Had that been the message from my papà, letting me know he was okay and I wasn't alone? A calm came over me as the barrier lifted, and I drove through. In that one moment, I knew he was still with me.

BACK WHEN I HAD GOTTEN My own tickets to see *The Phantom of the Opera*, I had bought another pair and gifted them to my parents for their wedding anniversary. The date for the performance they were to see was to be just after the New Year. I had planned to add to their experience with a gift certificate to some downtown restaurant that I would give them for Christmas. That way, Papà and Mamma could enjoy dinner and a show on me.

It had never once occurred to me when buying them that my papà would die before being able to use those tickets.

When the time neared, Mamma didn't want to go. No surprise. True to her Sicilian traditions, she wore black and mourned her husband's death. Christmas had been canceled for our whole family. She barely uttered more than a few words to anyone only if absolutely necessary. Most days, she slept, which was partly due to her grief but also due to the fact that she'd finally started taking her meds again, religiously, and they made her sleepy.

After I told Rosario Mamma's conspiracy theory warnings had started up again, he'd come over and made it very clear to her that he wasn't Papà, and he wouldn't put up with her non-compliance with her doctor's orders. He had bought her a pill organizer, and as he carefully counted and distributed all of her medications into each day's morning and evening compartments, he told her that at the first sign of her crazy rearing its ugly head, he would have her committed for life.

Mamma had taken his threat to heart, believing that he meant it, even though I knew he didn't. He was much more of a marshmallow than he would have liked to admit.

My brother didn't want to be the one to take Mamma to the theater, but she insisted that it was the only way she would agree to see *The Phantom of the Opera*.

"*Papà non c'è più, ed è giusto che mio figlio mi accompagnia.*"

I couldn't argue with Mamma's wishes. Papà was gone, and for her only son to accompany her, whether he wanted to or not, was right. Rosario knew it, too, and finally agreed.

Part of me thought I should just sell the tickets and recoup my money. Instead of a gift, it now felt as something being forced on people, more of a burden than anything else. Mamma, I was sure, would return from the musical as her usual stoic self. I would have bet money on it.

THE NIGHT OF THE SHOW, from my seat on the couch in the living room, the very place where Papà sat up late nights waiting for his daughter to come home after a night out with friends, I heard hurried footsteps making their way upstairs from the garage to where I waited. I turned off the TV and turned my body to greet my brother and mother.

Upon reaching the top of the landing, Mamma turned her head in my direction. Her coal-like eyes, usually devoid of expression, were sparkling and alive. She seemed thunderstruck, trying to catch her breath, as she approached me. Her entire face beamed.

"*Madonna, che bello!*" With every step Mamma took, she emphasized her words: "*B-E-A-U-T-I-F-U-L, Paola. Ti dico è stato Bellissimo!*"

I couldn't believe her reaction.

Who in the world is this, and what happened to Mamma?

It had been so long since I had seen any spark of life in Mamma. To see her this elated had me at a loss for words.

"You liked it?" I stammered.

"I love!" Mamma said as she wrapped her arms around me, hugging me so tightly that I couldn't help but hug her back.

Looking over her shoulder at Rosario, who had come upstairs right behind her, I raised my eyebrows.

"Pretty cool," he said, smiling, with a nod and a shrug.

I wasn't sure if he meant the musical or our mother's burst back to life.

When Mamma finally broke free from me, she stripped off her coat and took a seat in the recliner—Papà's favorite chair—and began to relive *The Phantom of the Opera*, sharing, scene by scene, in great detail, every single one of her favorite parts.

"*Il lampadario che oscilla con il fantasma nel pubblico . . . Spettacolare!*"

Recounting the chandelier scene when the Phantom swings into the audience left her breathless. Like a wind-up toy, Mamma radiated pure joy and excitement, with no sign of ever slowing down.

I could have listened to her for hours, days, months, years—for all the time that this Mamma had gone dormant. Somewhere inside of me, as much as I had given up on the hope that her health would improve, I had secretly dreamed of a moment like this for so long.

As part of me basked in her glow, however, another part questioned if she would have had this same reaction to the musical if Papà were still alive and had been the one to go with her. Had his candle burned so bright that she couldn't help but blow out her own?

I wondered.

CHAPTER SIXTEEN: **CRUISE CONTROL**

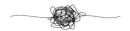

ROSARIO AND CATERINA HAD TAKEN me to my first concert when I was twelve years old. Styx's Grand Illusion tour had
come to the Rosemont Horizon, and they had surprised me for
my birthday with tickets on the main floor. Mamma had already
been deep into her madness by then, but we three were just
normal teenage siblings on that night. As I stood on my chair,
singing along to "Fooling Yourself" while Rosario held my hand,
making sure I wouldn't fall, we were together, connected, and I
felt so safe and free.

Fourteen years later, that was no longer the case. We each had
retreated into our own worlds. The aftershock of Papà's death
had split us apart, leaving me in the house alone with Mamma
and Viny. "Free" was the last thing I felt, and "escape" was the
thing for which I prayed.

While pretending got easier with practice, faking that everything was okay was still exhausting. Late one night, as I left work,
my coworker Sylvia, who managed the newspaper's special sections, asked if I wanted to grab dinner. She and I had never really
socialized outside of work before. I assumed it was because we
had little in common other than our jobs and our mutual love
for storytelling. Although just a few years older than me, Sylvia
was already married and was expecting her first baby any day.

To me, she looked like a carefree kid herself, way too young to be a mamma. Petite and pretty, with golden brown locks and a freckled face that was quick to smile, she, like I, worked long hours. Rarely, if ever, did she show signs of stress.

I agreed, and we headed out together to a nearby restaurant. As we ate, I started to share what I had never told her or anyone at the newspaper before.

"My mom's a paranoid schizophrenic," I blurted out.

"Oh, wow," Sylvia said. "I had no idea."

I went on to share my life of madness, spilling everything I had kept secret for so long. I told her about growing up with Mamma sitting in the living room at night screaming and swearing at who knows what for hours. I told her of the misdiagnoses and multiple brain surgeries, and of the struggles to fund treatments. I told her about having to take care of her and my little sister, especially now with my dad having died. I talked about Viny, and her not being able to do anything for herself. I shared about the screaming matches she used to have with our dad and was now having with me. I shared it all.

For hours, I talked and she listened. And when I had finished, she said, with tears in her eyes, "Oh my God. Me too."

Now it was my turn to listen and hers to talk: a dad who went from being an alcoholic to a paranoid alcoholic, often cussing to no one, just as Mamma did; a mom who drank; and a sister who battled her own demons. Sylvia had taken on the role of caregiver and was dealing with dysfunctional family crazy similar to what I faced at home.

For a moment, we both just looked at one another. I felt such a jolt of energy in the realization that here was one person who totally understood the madness surrounding me. I could see in her face that she felt the same way, too.

That night, getting into my car, driving back home, I thought about the connection I had found with this soul sister. What were the odds of us having such similar experiences and for Sylvia to show up just when I needed to not feel so alone?

As I drove past the cemetery, I waved at Papà from the road.

It was too late and dark to visit. A song started playing on the radio. I had never heard it before. Such a haunting sound and lyrics that sent a shock through my core: the singer crooned that although he'd died, he hadn't gone anywhere—that his loved one just had to think of him, and he'd be there. They announced the artists: The Escape Club. I laughed as tears welled up in my eyes. I wasn't alone. Far from it.

I WORRIED THAT THINGS WOULD be awkward with Sylvia at work now. I still didn't want anyone else to know about my life at home. To me, the more people who knew your weaknesses, the more you put yourself at risk of having your secrets used against you. I was relieved that Sylvia felt the same way. Like me, she had gotten quite good at hiding the madness in her life. In the end, it actually became easier, not more difficult, to be around one another and to be ourselves.

I wasn't sure if Sylvia was the one who told Karin how much I loved Rod Stewart, or if maybe I had blurted it out at some point. But when I learned that the newspaper was a major sponsor of his upcoming concert at Rosemont Horizon and I begged for tickets, Karin said okay.

For weeks, I told everyone who would listen that I had VIP tickets to see Rod Stewart. I would be "doo-wopping on stage" is what I actually ran around telling people, including Mamma. Not that I expected her to know who Rod Stewart even was.

"*Mi piace come canta*," Mamma said.

I tilted my head quizzically. "You like how he sings?" I was sure Mamma was mistaken. No way did she know who he was.

She insisted, nodding, and then began to sing: "If you want my body, I am very sexy."

I howled at Mamma's rendition of Rod Stewart's "Do Ya Think I'm Sexy." I applauded her as she blushed, giggling. I thought about Beth's mom, who'd danced in the bar in Iowa and whose favorite song Beth had known.

I asked Mamma if that was her favorite song.

She shook her head. "*Mi piace meglio quello che parla di la mamma.*"

She preferred one that talked about a mom? I wasn't sure which song she meant.

Mamma began to sing: "Mamma, I kill one man. No cry, Mamma . . ." They were the only words she knew, but they were enough. I took over, doing my best to sing the first few lines of my favorite band's operatic rock song. I barely got through the first stanza before Mamma recognized it and came alive.

Enthusiastically nodding, she almost shouted, "*Si, si! Come si chiama?*"

I answered her question, telling her the name of what I now knew was Mamma's favorite song—"Bohemian Rhapsody."

I'd always thought Mamma and I had nothing in common; maybe, I was wrong. And maybe what we did have in common had nothing to do with the voices.

IT HAD BEEN MORE THAN a year since Papà had died. I had again started dreaming of moving out on my own. It seemed possible. Mamma was better, taking her meds and not talking to or seeing things that weren't really there. Viny, on the other hand, was always going to be Viny. She did absolutely nothing to help out around the house. She barely came out of her room, other than to eat or go to her job.

I marched down the hall toward her bedroom one day as she followed, screaming, "Don't you go into my room, Pauley!"

"Vince, I told you not to take that job at the dry cleaners, didn't I?" I shouted at her. She'd had a job she could actually do, rolling silverware into napkins at Bishop's Buffet. But she'd quit in order to take a job that there was no way she could actually do. Steaming, pressing, folding, hanging? Viny couldn't even figure out how to put a dress on a hanger, let alone clean and iron one. But she refused to listen. She had become so strong-willed, almost delusional, convinced of her own grandeur.

I pushed open the door to her bedroom. It looked as if a

bomb had hit. It was worse than a teenager's room, with clothes strewn on the floor and papers with scribbles and drawings that looked like they belonged to a five-year-old littering the top of her dresser. Half-eaten bags of junk food and more of I don't know what could be seen stashed under her bed.

"Oh, my God!" I barked. "This is a disaster."

"It's my room!"

"Well now that you got fired from the cleaners, you've got time to clean this mess up."

"You don't understand," Viny cried. "My boss hit me."

"What? Why?" I asked as I looked around, wondering if it was safe to touch anything or if I needed a hazmat suit.

"She said I burned somebody's shirt. But I didn't."

I had no doubt Viny actually had ruined someone's clothes. And while her boss had no right to hit her, there were times I wanted to hit Viny, too. I probably would have raised a hand to her right then and there, but my anger lost its fuel when I saw the sliver of paper that sat on her nightstand.

"I'm a no talent bumb!" Viny's scribbly handwriting underscored the words expressing how she felt. "Can't get no job. Keep one once I get it. Either I go away or do nothing."

Her self-loathing note forced me to soften my tone.

"She shouldn't have hit you, Vince." I turned to face her, the runt of our litter. She was a carbon copy of what Mamma had looked like as a child, with her jet black hair and round, haunting eyes. Had it not been for those near-identical traits, I would have sworn Viny was switched at birth in the hospital. Nothing else about her seemed to fit in with the rest of us.

DR. LESSEN'S CLASS STRESSED THAT people with disabilities should be thought of as being exceptional. A disability was just an inability to do something. It didn't mean a person was incapable of doing *everything*. There was *something* everyone was good at doing.

In Viny's case, I had no idea what that could possibly be. There was only one thing she knew better than anyone I had ever met or even seen on TV, and that was music. She could hear the first few notes of a song on the radio and immediately know the title, the artist, and all of the lyrics.

She reminded me of Dustin Hoffman's character Raymond in the movie *Rain Man*. Raymond is a savant with a capacity to recall numbers, including baseball statistics. His brother Charlie, a character played by Tom Cruise—seeing Raymond's innate talent and how helpful it might be to the gambler in him—gets Raymond a "job" counting cards in blackjack. Granted, it's illegal, but Charlie does find the one thing his brother can do and puts it to work.

The one thing Viny could do didn't seem to open up any career options, though, legal or illegal. At least, none that I could figure out. And she couldn't seem to learn much of how to do anything else that she *could* apply to her daily life.

The Pioneer Center she was frequenting for socialization and empowerment had said they offered vocational services. That translated into two words Viny refused to even consider: job coach. The more I tried to push her into it, the more belligerent and unmanageable she became.

Wanting her to engage in something, anything, I assigned her more chores to do around the house. Mowing the lawn was one I figured she could handle, until I came home to see her first attempt at it had proven she could not. The lawn looked like a mish-moshed maze, with grass left untouched in some spots and completely dug up in others. It was as if she had run the mower over and over the same bald spot until all that remained was dirt.

By the very next weekend, that task had reverted back to me.

On the days I did the grocery shopping, I dreaded the battle that awaited me when I got home with bags to unload from my trunk.

"Viny!" I would scream from the garage door, calling for her to come help me take the groceries upstairs to the kitchen and put them away. She moved slower than a sloth. And if she saw something I had purchased that interested her, she'd eat it all in one sitting or use it in some self-created recipe that would have Mamma and me gagging.

"You're just jealous!" Viny would scream. "I can cook better than both of you."

Taking care of Mamma and Viny, figuring out their disability and social security and other government filings, dealing with hospitals, doctor visits, and medical bills, managing the household, working a full-time job, and doing most everything by myself . . . at twenty-seven years old, I felt closer to eighty.

My weight, approaching the 300-pound mark, wasn't helping. Nor was the fact that I rarely socialized in bars or dance clubs like normal single women my age. My routine was home to work, work to home, and any in-between time was spent eating and watching TV or going to the movies.

Occasionally, I still visited Papà's grave, but it no longer brought comfort; rather, it only reminded me of the role that was my fate, and that I now fully owned. His beautiful garden had pretty much filled in. Gone were its ruby red rows of ripe plum tomatoes, its fragrant blooms of basil, its purple pear-shaped eggplant, its five-foot-long, trumpet-like zucchini. Now all that remained, as if in tribute to what once was, was the solitary soldier of a grape vine. Having come of age, its branches were now all gnarled and twisted, and it fought a never-ending battle against the vicious weeds that surrounded and choked its roots. It clung to life, pinned against that old wire fence, a lonely sentinel that continued to bear fruit: plump clusters of sweet, thin-skinned, champagne-colored grapes—yearly reminders of what my Papà had lovingly labored for but never gotten to taste.

I could barely look at what I had failed to maintain; I hated coming home to it day after day.

WHEN SYLVIA ASSIGNED ME TO a story featuring a local fitness center and spa that catered only to women for the newspaper's Health & Fitness special section, I thought twice about accepting it. How would it look with someone as big as me coming in to interview physically fit Chicagoans? Would anyone believe I was capable of writing a credible story? I finally understood Mamma's concerns about appearances.

As I walked into The Women's Club and roamed around the main areas, I saw so many normal-size (at least compared to me) women huffing and puffing on the treadmills and dancing in the aerobics classes. Immediately, I regretted saying yes to writing the article.

A woman walked toward me, hand extended for a shake. "Hi, I'm Margie," she said. "I'm the owner of The Women's Club."

I searched her eyes as I shook her hand, bracing myself for what I fully expected to see in them: disgust at the body that housed me.

How could someone like you even begin to appreciate, let alone communicate, what her center has to offer?

What a loser, a big fat loser.

To my surprise, however, I saw nothing but kindness in Margie's bright eyes. They matched her hair's fiery shade of amber. She was probably in her forties but looked much younger and so very pretty. Not model pretty—more like tomboy cute.

We clicked. For the next couple of hours, we talked about her and her fitness center and spa. And for longer than that, we talked about things beyond The Women's Club. Before I knew it, not only had the story already written itself, but Margie had also offered me a free membership in exchange for interviewing club members and putting together some promotional testimonial ads.

I committed to coming in to exercise at least three days each week. The Club was just a few miles from the newspaper, and on the way home, so I had no excuses.

AS IT TURNED OUT, I DIDN'T need any excuses—I enjoyed going to the gym. It wasn't so much a desire to move my body and sweat as it was a love for the spa's whirlpool. It became my reward for working out, and sometimes the only thing I would end up doing there. The feel of being weightless was one I had never had before and could get nowhere else.

While Margie hadn't a clue about my home life, she seemed to zero in on my need to take better care of myself.

I knew it, too. I needed a break from Mamma and Viny and caring for everybody other than me. So when Donna suggested that we go on a cruise to the Caribbean, I didn't hesitate to ask for the time off from my job.

Unfortunately, the cruise I could afford launched on Mother's Day. Tremendous guilt set in when I realized I wouldn't be around for Mamma on her special day. But I asked her permission; would she mind if I went?

"*Vai, vai, divertite!*" Mamma echoed some of the last words Papà had said to me, encouraging me to go and have fun.

I booked the cruise and couldn't wait to go.

For the next few months, I felt such giddiness. Wrapped up in my own happiness and excitement, I barely took note when Viny started corresponding with some boy via the personal ads. A Sicilian boy, she said. They had struck up a phone relationship and it had been going on for several weeks now, she said. I didn't question it. I barely acknowledged it.

I raced to finish my projects at work so I could feel completely free while on my cruise. As special thanks to Mamma for giving the green light to me being away on Mother's Day, I wrote a Mother's Day column for the newspaper and set it up in the queue to publish on Sunday, May 10, 1992, as a surprise for her.

The headline the editor set to kick off my piece would read, "Tragedy Lets Her See Mother In New Light," and the column I would share with readers was my silver lining story: how close I had been to my papà; how lost I'd felt when he died; and how much I was enjoying getting to know my mamma.

I closed with, "Although things will never be the same *without* my dad, it makes me happy to know that things will never be the same *with* my mom."

WHEN THE DAY TO START my vacation finally came, I raced around the house last-minute packing. To make it to Chicago's O'Hare Airport to catch an 8:30 a.m. flight to Miami meant I had to be on the road by 6:00 a.m. Already behind when I should have left the house, I had no time to spare.

With my bags zipped up, I said my good-byes to Mamma, kissing her and telling her I would call on Mother's Day. She kissed me back and told me to behave myself. Carrying my luggage toward the stairs, I yelled out a good-bye to Viny, who was still in her bedroom. I had just taken the first few steps heading downstairs to the garage when Viny appeared, standing in the hallway, barely visible at the top of the stairs, almost as if she was trying to hide herself from being noticed or fully coming forth.

"Pauley, can I talk to you?" Her voice trembled.

I pretended not to notice and continued on my way. "Vince, I really gotta go or I won't make my flight."

"Just two minutes? It's important."

I purposely didn't look at my sister. "No, I gotta go. You do this every time. Every time I do something for me. No. Not this time. We can talk when I get back."

I dragged my bags downstairs and into the garage, and then slammed the door behind me. Having cruelly dismissed her, I imagined Viny still standing there at the top of the stairs, her chin quivering, the tears in her eyes threatening to spill over.

Something inside me knew. "It" was trying to tell me that "it" was coming. History was about to repeat itself. I just wasn't paying attention. And even if a tiny part of me did have a clue, the rest of me didn't want to hear it.

ON BOARD THE CRUISE SHIP, we set sail for the Western Caribbean. Donna directed our schedule, and I followed. On the first day, she wanted to go down to the ship's theatre to play bingo.

"I hate bingo, Donna," I said, dragging my feet.

"Come on, it'll be fun!" she exclaimed.

Grumpily, I sat next to her in the seats high up and toward the back. With my bingo paper packs and dauber at the ready, I listened to the cruise director yell out numbers, not really understanding much of his code.

"A deck of cards," he shouted out.

"Fifty-two!" Donna excitedly answered the riddles, leaning over to make sure I didn't miss any numbers on my cards.

"This is so lame," I complained.

"Life begins at . . ." Another number called out.

"Forty!" Donna bounced in her chair like a little kid as I rolled my eyes.

Number after number, I begrudgingly played. And then, all of a sudden, looking down at one of my sheets, I heard myself yell out, "BINGO!!"

"We have a winner!" the announcer proclaimed as the spot lights shined in my direction.

Donna applauded and hooted like an owl, celebrating my win.

"Beginner's luck." I shrugged, feeling a bit sheepish. I had fought her for much of the way down to play the game, and yet here I was now, pocketing the prize of $110. It didn't seem fair.

On Day Two, Mother's Day, I took time out to telephone Mamma ship to shore. One minute cost $15, but with my winnings, I could afford at least five.

Our chat was brief; mostly, it was me talking. I told her that the midnight buffet said it included *cappelletti*, but that I knew there was no way they'd taste as great as hers. Mamma laughed and told me to enjoy and be happy.

I never once thought about talking to Viny, or even asking about her.

The following days' cruising included shopping excursions in Cozumel, sunbathing on the white sandy beaches of Grand Cayman, ordering up double desserts and sometimes even entrees during dinners, and completely vegging out on the deckchairs during our days at sea while what we called "cabana boys" served us boozy drinks in oversized mason jars. Night after night, we returned to our cabin no earlier than 2:00 a.m., and still stayed up hours longer, fantasizing about making it with one of the wait staff or crew members.

This was better than normal. I hadn't a care in the world and didn't care if I ever went back home.

CHAPTER SEVENTEEN: **CRAZY**

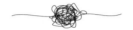

AND THEN, I WAS HOME.

And for the tiniest bit of time, nothing felt the same, but in a good way. The air smelled cleaner. The sun shined brighter. Traffic flowed uncongested. Even stopping at Papà's grave didn't produce a single tear; I smiled as I updated him on my trip and the souvenirs I had brought home for Mamma and Viny. Any thought of what had happened before I had left home for the cruise had been wiped clean of my memory. The seven days away had freed me from the weight of responsibilities and obligations. I had probably gained another 20 pounds during my vacation, and yet I felt at least that much lighter.

By the time I pulled up into the driveway and clicked the remote to automatically raise our home's garage door, I couldn't wait to see Mamma and Viny. While still in the car, I caught Mamma peering out the front windows. I waved to her, but she didn't wave back. Instead, she quickly pulled back and out of view while I proceeded to drive into the garage and park.

A few minutes later, I dragged my luggage in through the front door. I was keeping one eye on the garage door to make sure it closed properly—and I nearly bumped foreheads with Mamma who was waiting for me just inside.

"*Paola, siamo mezz'i guai,*" she gasped, a look of horror on her face.

I dropped my suitcase and other bags. "What do you mean, 'We're in the middle of trouble'?"

My mother's breathing seemed on the verge of hyperventilation. Her eyes were hollowed-out black spheres, seemingly frozen in a state of surprise. She held her hands one in the other, kneading them raw. She looked as if she had not slept since I had left.

She had not.

"*Vincenzina . . .*" her voice trailed off. She hugged me, and I felt her body release as she began to sob.

"*Che c'è? Mamma? Che è successo??*" My mother's show of emotion unnerved me. I needed her to tell me now what happened.

"*Tutto la serata, gridi, piangere . . .*"

"Who was up all night yelling and crying?"

My sister Viny barreled out from the hallway and down the stairs to the entryway where Mamma and I stood.

"Pauley, you're home! You're not going to believe this!" she screeched, teetering between the second and third steps of our staircase.

She looked wild. Hair unkempt. Clothes disheveled. An almost halo effect surrounding her face, communicating crazy through those eyes that mimicked Mamma's. Her entire being screamed *savage*; it was as if she had seen the second coming of Christ or the resurrection of Papà.

It should have hit me then. But it didn't. Not entirely. I think I was in shock. There's a fine line between experiencing, knowing, and accepting. And it took me a moment to gather up the courage to cross the chasm of crazy. Again.

Yet another shoe dropping. This time, Viny.

I heard myself—not the voices in my head but my own voice, but from afar, as if I had stepped outside of myself to address her: "What's wrong, Vince?"

"Wrong? Nothing's wrong. That's so like you to think everything with me is wrong."

The rage in her mounted.

"It's not always the good things that happen only to you, you know. And for your information, I'm engaged." My sister sported a terrifying smile that frightened me.

"Engaged?"

"Yes, engaged. What? Is that so hard to believe?"

"No," I was feeling myself becoming more and more afraid, from the inside out. "No, Vince, it's just that I've never heard of a guy, I mean—"

"I wanted to tell you but nooo, you had to leave on your trip. Well, too bad! I'm getting married before you. His name is Costante—"

"*No, Vincenzinamia; non è possibile,*" my mother squeaked, insisting weakly that it wasn't possible.

"It iiiiissssss possible!" Viny hissed, raising up on her tiptoes and screaming.

"Okay, Vince, okay."

At that moment, I knew. Schizophrenia had made its choice on who to possess next.

"So who is this guy? When do we get to meet him?"

"I'll call him right now. He's so great. Just you wait. It'll happen to you, too, one day!"

My sister climbed the stairs, faster than I had ever seen her move before, and disappeared into Mamma's back bedroom.

"Oh, Paola!" Mamma climbed the stairs.

Leaving my luggage behind, I followed, watching as she dragged herself to Papà's old chair in the living room, slumped down into it, and put her head in her hands.

I stood there for a moment. How I wished Papà was still here. And how glad I was that he wasn't.

Part of me realized immediately that the very midnight screaming I had experienced in my youth as Mamma battled her demons all night long was now being experienced firsthand by Mamma herself as she witnessed the same demons lashing out from inside her youngest daughter. Papà didn't need to deal with that again. None of us did. For Mamma, however, this experience was a first and had to be worse than even I could imagine.

Instinctively, I wanted to hug her; I could not help but feel her pain, and I wanted to take it away. While Viny was in a very real way *our* daughter, given how I had helped raise her when Mamma could not, I had the luxury of stepping back and shunning any real responsibility if I chose to. I was just her sister. Mamma, however, had no choice but to claim her offspring and bear the burden of knowing that she was the one to have passed on her insanity genes and this terrifying mental illness.

I snapped to when I heard Viny screaming, "You let me talk to him; he's my fiancé!"

I raced into the kitchen to pick up the receiver of the other phone. I listened in as a male voice—older, gruff, angered—said, "You listen to me. I don't know what this is, but my son wants nothing to do with you. And if you don't stop harassing him, I'm going to call the police!"

Instinct kicked in: "Excuse me. My name is Paolina. I'm Viny's sister. Who is this?"

"This is Costante's father. Your sister won't leave my son alone. I think there's something wrong with her—"

"There's nothing wrong with me!" Viny screamed into the phone. "You're just trying to keep us apart!"

I spoke in as soothing a voice as I could muster: "Okay, okay. Viny calm down. Sir, I think there may be something wrong. I'm very sorry for the trouble. I ask that you don't call the police. I'll get my sister some help."

Viny slammed down the phone and began screaming in the other room. The boy's father agreed, saying he hoped my sister would be okay. I barely heard him when Viny came storming down the hall to where I was.

"How could you do that to me? You're just jealous!"

"Viny, Viny listen to me—"

"No. No. I'm not listening to anyone anymore! I'll show you. You'll see." She stormed back to her bedroom.

I walked behind her but then chose to go down the stairs to get my luggage that I had left just inside the front door. As I was dragging my suitcases backwards back up the stairs, I had barely reached the third step when my sister, screaming, started heading from her bedroom down the hall back toward me. I spun around, let go of my bags, and planted both feet on the same stair, willing myself not to move. Something inside me told me that to flinch even an inch would result in my sister killing me.

Viny barreled down the stairs. She raised both fists, her face a storm of darkness and evil, her eyes daggers of hate and rage. She came at me and only stopped when she was within a centimeter of my face. I did not move, barely breathed, and stared her down. With one final, ear-piercing scream, her nose brushing mine, she pushed me aside and ran out the door.

This can't be happening.

Swallowing to catch my breath, I turned to follow her out the door—and then reversed directions and ran back upstairs into the kitchen, where I picked up the phone and dialed my brother.

His voicemail picked up. I waited for the beep.

"Ross, can you please come home? Something's wrong with Viny. It's the same thing as Mamma. Please come." My voice broke. I hung up.

I took a deep breath and forced myself to shake it off.

Mamma hovered by, pacing and wringing her hands. I couldn't look at her. Instead, I made my way down the hall to Viny's room.

I opened the door to an entire room littered with sheets of paper, all different colors and sizes, some crumpled, some straight and smooth, all with writing on them. Pages and pages and hundreds of letters written by someone so lost, so angry, so not my little sister. Picking a few up, I began to read.

"You better do as I say or you and your family will pay."

My blood turned to ice as I read the words Viny had written. My mind forced me to revisit the time a few years earlier when I'd been watching TV and had become mesmerized by the news unfolding of that woman named Laurie Dann. Visions of her dark hair and black-hole eyes, which so closely mimicked Viny's features, filled my head. The two could be sisters.

But you're her sister.

"I know!" I shouted, without intending to.

Mamma who had followed me, standing in the doorway, jumped, the crooked fingers of her right hand pressing against her temple. "*Che c'è?*"

I couldn't answer Mamma, because I couldn't even begin to make sense of all the thoughts competing to be heard as I read Viny's letters.

"Instead of horseplay, I'll be more severe. I hope this is clear to all of you. There'll be so much pain that either of you even in your wildest dreams ever knew could exist."

I raised a hand to my own head. One week ago—just seven days ago—had all of this been here? Had I missed it? Had crazy—for the second time—come calling and slipped in the back door, determined yet again to stay?

I read more. Viny's last few lines raged with the intent to, quite possibly, do what Laurie Dann had done.

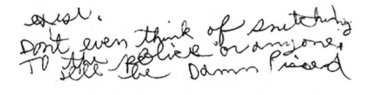

"Don't even think of snitching to the police or anyone. I'll be damn pissed."

The voices in my head scolded me loudly.

And you would be one of the family members interviewed who'd say something stupid like "she was so normal," when you knew damn well she wasn't. Ever.

They needed to shut up. I needed to think.

"Paola, che faciamo?" My mother still stood just outside the bedroom door, asking me what we were going to do.

Mamma needed to shut up too. I just couldn't deal with what was happening. I ignored her, lost in the letters I had found. How could I have been soaking in the sun, lying on sugared beaches in the calm of the Caribbean, just days ago? Had that really happened? Was this really happening?

I no longer knew what was or wasn't real.

Another letter shattered my frozen heart.

> give me something for
> this pain.
>
> So I can laugh, smile, be
> happy again.
>
> all I've known is fear
> + terror.
> I'd like to be like others who never
> complain.

"*Give me something for this pain.*"

"Paola?" Mamma begged.

I could not stand to hear my mother's voice. I could not stand to see one more scribbling, one more shred of evidence that would shine a light on what I knew we were in for: History repeating itself in the worst of ways. Yet I kept reading.

> You endanger everyone you touch.
> even the ones who care, and love
> you so much.
> you don't care about anyone but
> yourself.

"*You endanger everyone you touch . . .*"

I struggled to read more, wondering now which messages were directed at whom. She had wanted to tell me something before I had left on my trip. I hadn't had time for her, couldn't be bothered.

your only wish is to save your own hide, as long as your satisfied.
nothing else matters, you could care less if others are hurt or their dreams and passions are shattered.

You didn't care about her dreams.
All she wanted was for you to listen. Why didn't you?
You're partly to blame for this.

Its of no importance when there's blood shed and all are dead.

The words on the page grew in size—"*blood shed*" and "*dead*"—seeming to leap off the page.

"*Paola, per favore . . .*" My mother begged for a response, for guidance; she, too, was lost.

Shut up, shut up, shut up, the voices shouted.

I so wanted to scream with them.

I changed my mind. I wished Papà was there. I wanted to snap back to my mother, "I don't know what to do!" But I stayed silent.

Because I did know.

I knew exactly what needed to be done. And in that moment, a switch was flipped inside of me. Robotically, I set forth to do what I had to do, what I had seen my papà do years before, and from somewhere within me, I thanked him for lessons well taught.

"ST. JOSEPH'S HOSPITAL, HOW may I direct your call?" The operator on the other end of the telephone asked. The receiver felt sweaty as my hand gripped it. I tried to quiet the tremors inside as I leaned against the refrigerator in the kitchen, supporting myself, feeling as if I was ready to fall.

"Psychiatric ward, please." I waited to be connected.

The voice on the other end needed little detail. I explained the situation. I was advised to capture my sister and bring her to the emergency room. They would be waiting.

I hung up the phone, found my keys, and told Mamma that I would be back. I set forth to search for a sister I hoped was not so lost she could not ever be found.

Miraculously, before I even pulled out of the driveway, I saw my brother racing my way.

He immediately parked his truck in the driveway, got out, and climbed into the passenger side of my Ford Escort.

"What happened?" he demanded.

I explained.

Denial.

Clearly, he said, I had gotten it wrong. I had misunderstood. I was overreacting and being dramatic. There was "no way," he said, that this was happening again.

I stayed silent and prayed I really was wrong.

Soon, we saw Viny nearly skipping along the sidewalk, carrying with her what looked like pamphlets and brochures. We stopped the car. Ross exited and pulled his seat forward.

"Come on, Vince, get in."

She did. "Ross, look; Pauley doesn't believe me, but it's all over the place. See?" She handed him the papers.

We drove off.

"What am I looking at?" My brother's face started as a mask of confusion and then slowly turned to a shield of fearful realization.

"Look!" Viny screamed, half laughing, half crying. "These are stories about me. My upcoming wedding. See the picture of me and Costante? Aren't we beautiful together?"

I glanced over at the pamphlets—church bulletins and shopping circulars she had picked up from somewhere. The pictures were of no one we knew; most weren't even of people but rather of products being promoted. I turned my eyes back to the road ahead, to the beacon of hope I sought in the form of the hospital.

Suddenly, my brother erupted, slamming his fist onto the dashboard, causing me to jump. "This isn't you, Viny," he growled. "These aren't stories or pictures of you, and there is no wedding!"

Viny sobbed. "You don't believe me, like Paula. You're trying to keep me down."

I must have been channeling Papà and his years of experience: "Vince, it's not that we don't believe you. We're actually gonna go right now to a counselor to help us understand better and make preparations for you and Costante and your wedding."

"Really? Oh, thank you. I really love you guys. And you can be in the wedding. Will you be my maid of honor?"

"Sure, Vince. Sure."

Ross and I exchanged looks of dread, looks of knowing. We drove the rest of the way in silence while Viny chatted on to others—an entire bridal party of friends whom she believed to be in the car with us.

We stopped in front of the emergency room doors. Ross exited and helped Viny out from the backseat. We entered the hospital. I gave my name. They knew what to do.

So did I.

On May 16, 1992, I committed my twenty-four-year-old little sister to a psych ward. As if it was the most natural thing to do, even as I wrote my signature on so many legal documents, my hand barely shook, never once wavered. It, too, knew what to do, almost as if it didn't need me to tell it.

"We'll take good care of your sister. Don't worry. You're doing the right thing."

The nurse behind the desk in the emergency room of St. Joseph's Hospital patted my hand. She then held on to it, as it suddenly started to shake to the point that I struggled with the pen. All I needed to do was to sign my name on the line at the bottom of the last page. That's all it would take to finish committing my baby sister to a psych ward. But the pen refused to stay steady between my fingers.

THIS is anything but normal.

And yet I should have known. If not when she was a kid, then all throughout her teenage years, her adulthood . . .

The nurse released my hand. "Hon, we need your final signature to be able to start treating your sister."

I forced my hand to place the tip of the pen on the line where I was to sign. In a weird déjà vu that I would wish on no one, I recalled watching my own papà sign Mamma's commitment papers at least a decade earlier. Now I watched my own hand, as if completely detached from me, sign my own name, taking the lead role this time in locking away a member of my family. I shut my eyes and finished scribbling my name.

Ross and I stood side by side in complete silence.

I had taken on the role of caregiver for my sister long ago, as soon as Mamma had fallen victim to schizophrenia, back when I was about ten. As Ross and I moved like zombies to sit and wait in the hospital lobby to talk to someone, anyone, about Viny's fate, I took on all the blame and guilt. Again, if anybody should have seen the signs, clearly, it was me.

"Ms. Milana?"

Ross and I turned in the direction the voice had come from. A white coat–clad man with a clipboard, chart, and pen in hand waved us over. We rose from our seats and proceeded to meet him.

He shook my hand and Ross's and guided us to a little room with television monitors. He told us his name, but I was too fixated on what I saw on the TVs: my little sister, Viny, in a bare-bones room, the walls padded, not much more than a bed in its center, having a conversation with—whom, I wasn't quite sure. No one else was in the picture, and yet she was arguing and responding and laughing at jokes with whomever else she believed was there.

"Your sister is experiencing paranoid delusions," he said. "We've got her in our 'quiet room' for observation and to get her to calm down. She'll be safe here."

I watched Viny on the monitor. She cried out and raged against no one. She switched to knee-slapping laughter and wide-eyed, top-of-her-lungs singing. She seemed at home in her surroundings, as if in her own bedroom, only to snap into a fit of fear, begging to be let out, calling for Ross or me to come save her.

My core felt as if, cell by cell, it was disintegrating. I needed to sit.

"Please don't worry." The man in the white coat said empathetically with a hint of authority. "We see this a lot. This is perfectly normal behavior."

Rosario and I exchanged glances.

As normal as it was, it wasn't. And I, for one, hated that it had become our normal.

CHAPTER EIGHTEEN: **COMMITTED**

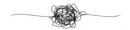

MY BROTHER AND I DID NOT SPEAK during the car ride home. How could this be happening to us again? My mind raced, shocked.

We parked in the driveway. Mamma stood just inside the front door. Her ghostly face and horrified eyes peered out at us as we exited the car. She could wait no more. Easing the door open and stepping outside in her housecoat and slippers, she called out in a quivering voice, "*Ma, Vincenzina, dov'è?*"

I guessed she may already know the answer—but even so, how was I supposed to respond? How could I tell Mamma that we'd left Viny, her baby, in a psych ward, just like we had done to her so many years before?

Rosario's red face registered rage as he barked, "Inside!"

Mamma didn't move.

I slowly dragged my body up the three steps to where she stood. Nodding my head, I gently turned her around and nudged her back inside. We all made our way upstairs and into the living room.

I'd expected to feel the same about my little sister's institutionalization as I had about Mamma's madness growing up. When we committed Mamma, I'd been overjoyed. The thought of being free from the crazy even for a little while? I was all in. They could have kept Mamma for as long as they liked. So when I'd signed Viny away, almost as easily as signing a credit card receipt, and told myself I was doing what I had to do, I hadn't been prepared for the consequences. Now, I couldn't catch my breath. My insides seemed to be swelling to the point of rupture. Something seemed to be crushing me from the inside out.

Nothing to see here.

I talked myself down: *Keep it together.* I simply had to do what I had learned so well to do: pretend.

"*Paola, che è successo?*" Mamma wrung her hands, smoothing them one in the other while pacing. She always paced. Back and forth, back and forth—the beige of the carpet worn to streaks of dirty gray, the creaking of the floorboards beneath her repeat steps making my shoulders rise up to my ears. To me, the act and the accompanying sound were no different than what I imagined the constant drip of water torturing might be to some prisoner.

"*Mamma, per che non ti sedi?*" I invited my mother to sit as I myself took a seat on the couch.

"Let her pace!" Caterina's voice echoed down the hall and into the living room, with her following. "What happened? What did you do?"

Rosario pleaded, "*Siediti, Ma.*"

Mamma sat. She always seemed to do what my brother asked of her. Maybe because he was the only boy in the family. Or maybe it was because of how he asked.

Rosario got it. Sort of. Except when he didn't. Like when he'd say, "You're not paying rent, you sometimes have to take Ma and Viny somewhere, big deal. Quit being the martyr."

Caterina wanted to get it. But only if "it" was what she wanted to hear. "I'm part of this family, too. I have a right to know." She stood in the center of the room, wanting answers.

My head felt so heavy, in such a fog. What *had* happened? Had it really happened? Or had I overreacted to what was maybe not crazy but the result of a broken heart and stomped-on spirit? Hers and mine.

"Cathy, you weren't here. You didn't see . . ." I felt such a need to defend myself. Always.

I thought about saying the same thing—shut the fuck up—to her now that I'd said the night of Papà's heart attack. What I really needed was silence. I needed to think. Why wouldn't everyone just be quiet for a little bit? Stop asking questions. Stop wanting me to come up with the answers. *Please, please God, make the voices stop.*

"They have her in the quiet room," I started to explain.

"Why the hell is she there?"

It was as if my older sister had never been around this block before.

"Cathy, if you don't shut the fuck up and listen, I swear to God I will kill you." I couldn't help it. The words just came out on their own, and with my sister they flowed easily.

"*Per favore*, no fight." Mamma struggled to hold back tears. She rose from her chair to start her never-ending, soul-soothing pacing.

My shoulders rose to my ears again.

Why Cathy and I never seemed to be quite on the same page any longer was a mystery to me. Where was the sister who used to write me those letters? Why could I so easily forgive Rosario and make allowances for his choices, but not so much for her? Why did I expect more from her and Mamma, come to think of it, than I ever had from Ross or even Papà?

"*Che pensi? Chi abbia cambiato i pannolini per voi bambini? Papà non mi ha aiutato affatto finché mi sono ammalata.*" Mamma had spat this back at me shortly after Papà died, disclosing that she'd been the one to change our diapers—that Papà had never lifted a finger until she got sick.

Maybe I was the one who didn't get it. Any of it.

I explained as best I could the chain of events that resulted in my committing our youngest sibling to a mental hospital. Cathy wasn't buying it. I expected Ross to chime in, but he didn't. And I couldn't tell if it was because he, too, wasn't convinced yet or because he was too shocked beyond belief that this was happening to us again to participate in the conversation.

No, Cathy, we shouldn't have had a family meeting before locking her away.

No, Cathy, they won't let us in for two weeks.

I silently responded to my sister's questions, refusing to

answer aloud. It angered her more, but at that moment keeping my mouth shut gave me a bit of relief.

"*Paola, andiamo a vederla?*"

My brother finally found his voice. "*Ma, non possiamo.*"

"Well if we can't go see her, can we call and get updates?" Cathy's concern felt more accusatory, as if she wanted to follow up and make sure Viny's commitment was warranted.

"I think only Paula can; she signed her in." Rosario responded.

And there it was. I signed her in. I was responsible. I did it. I hadn't done what I should have prior to it escalating to this point, so it was my fault. I seemed to have the power to give life, stop death, keep crazy at bay. So it seemed everyone else thought. At times, I myself was convinced that this was true. Yet what they didn't know was that I felt like the most powerless person on the planet. Damned whether I did or didn't.

Scanning the room, my eyes happened to rest on the portrait of our family that hung on the wall above the piano. How many times had Papà asked me to play something for him? How many times had I refused? How many times had I played one of his favorite pieces perfectly?

How I missed my papà.

Mamma had thought she might die on the operating table during one of her brain surgeries. That's what had prompted the family portrait, back when I was in high school. She'd wanted to make sure we had one official picture to remember her by.

Not a one of us had wanted to take that photo. The morning of the shoot had been filled with fighting over what to wear, messing with our hair, and getting to the studio on time. Once there, however, the photographer had known just what to do: treat us like children. From the moment we walked in, he'd started telling jokes, pulling pranks, and playing peek-a-boo with a bunny to get us to look into the camera and smile. We'd had to stop a couple of times because Papà was laughing so hard, and he hadn't wanted to show off his lack of teeth. Even Mamma hadn't been able to help but giggle like a schoolgirl. We actually looked so normal—so happy— in the picture.

"*Oh, Ma, ti ho portato un regalo dalla nave per il giorno delle Mamme.*" I had suddenly noticed the two Mother's Day cards sitting on top of the piano. I had been on my cruise during that day, had forgotten about a card. I had gotten her a gift from the ship, however, and I blurted that fact out now, guiltily.

"A Mother's Day gift? Now? And you think *I'm* a bitch?" Cathy snorted.

I realized her point. Not great timing on my part.

"I'm going to bed," I announced. I needed silence. I needed sleep. I needed to be anywhere but there.

Miraculously, Ross and Cathy left without objecting.

As I lay in my bed that night, with my mother in hers across the hall, I felt compelled to shout out to her, "I love you, Ma."

I was surprised to hear the response, in English—words I had never before in my life heard from her.

"I love you, too, Paola."

I WAS TOSSING AND TURNING all night long. I should have known. I knew about Viny's isolation, her friendless existence. I saw her get bullied daily at school. I knew she had been forced to stay in the house alone with Mamma, day in and day out. I knew of and had witnessed firsthand her out of control anger rants and increasingly emboldened verbal fights with Papà. I knew that schizophrenia was hereditary, despite what the doctors continuously told us.

Somewhere deep within me, I'd known all along.

Better her than me.

Please, God, don't let it be in me.

There still was a chance. My constant prayer still needed to be said. I had three more years until I hit the magic age of thirty and would be free and clear from mental illness claiming me. Until then, the fact that it had chosen to take root in Viny did not mean it wouldn't want more.

Had I fallen far enough from the family tree?

I guess in my desire to not be one of schizophrenia's chosen ones, I'd never given thought to how I'd feel should one of my other siblings draw the short end of the stick. And I'd especially never considered how I'd feel if it was the sibling I'd helped raise and regarded more like my child than my sister. I'd never given thought to how I would feel. Never given thought to how she would feel.

I knew already what to expect with Viny's illness. As we'd learned from our continuing battle with Mamma's, insanity was a life sentence. Crazy came with its own never-ending story. In years past, I'd often tried to barter with God, accepting being the one chosen but praying for a substitute disease: cancer, inoperable tumors, you name it. Anything that brought with it an end—"You have six months to live," versus, "You have a mental illness that will go on forever and sometimes, if we get your meds right and if you take them religiously, you might experience moments of 'normal.'"

My little sister, who had once been so adorable, had grown up to be not so cuddly, and to live in a never-ending story of sickness. And like our mother, she'd kept it quiet, hidden, and so it had gone unnoticed or ignored for too long.

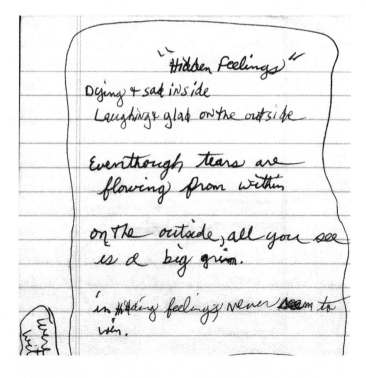

Just as it had been when we first committed Mamma to the hospital years before, for two weeks, we weren't allowed to visit Viny in the psych ward. During that time, I worked, pretending nothing was amiss. And when at home, I pored over more of her letters.

Don't want to be beat or hurt every time I turn around.
I'd like someone to know where I am so I can be found.
Before it's too late.

I prayed it wasn't too late.

Mamma begged for me to call for updates. I did. They pretty much just confirmed that she was confused and that they were medicating her.

When we were finally allowed to visit, we did, just as we had done before. We waited in a small conference room, all alone together. The sun streamed in from the window. We sat on little plastic chairs that were lined up against the wall. The door opened up and a nurse helped guide Viny across the threshold.

Disheveled and looking so much smaller than her usual size, as if deflated, like a balloon that had lost its helium, Viny immediately walked over to Ross and wrapped her arms around his waist.

"It's okay, Vince," he told her, and gently guided her to sit down in one of the chairs.

My heart was breaking seeing her like this. The crushing feeling in my chest made it uncomfortable to sit, so I stood. "How are you feeling?" I asked.

"Okay." Viny's eyes rolled around in her head.

"*Vincenzinamia*, be happy."

Mamma's favorite mantra: Be happy. I scoffed, although I had nothing better to say. And at least Mamma had said, "my Viny." I prayed it resonated with my sister.

"You don't belong here, Viny."

Caterina's words of wisdom only gave rise to my anger. I felt like asking her, "Okay, so should she come live with you?" But I exercised more restraint than was generally in my nature.

"I'm getting married," Viny said. "Did Pauley tell you?" While she was slurring her words, thanks to the number of drugs in her system, her convictions were clear.

"Vince, that guy doesn't want to see you. You're not getting married." Rosario. Again, always direct, even when the results might be disastrous.

I will never forget what came next. I have tried to expunge it from my memory, but I can't.

My sister sat in that chair. She heard our brother's words. She waited a moment. And then, like an infant, she threw back her head and, mouth open wide, screamed out a cry that no one could hear. Utter silence. Just the visual of her mouth open wide, her head back, her eyes shut, and nothing coming out.

Until something did.

And when it did, her cry was deafening. I found myself breathing out in short bursts, like a woman in labor, just to get through it.

"Viny, it's gonna be okay. I promise," I said, knowing I was lying—I didn't know if it was going to be okay—but unable to stop myself from saying it. I could not stand to see or hear her that way. I swallowed down tears.

I don't remember what came next. Maybe I wasn't paying attention. Maybe I was blocking it out. I just could not deal. This was my baby, my Viny. And I'd failed. I'd helped to fuck her up. Just as Mamma had us. Unknowingly.

BY DAY, I WENT TO WORK AT the newspaper. Sitting in my cubicle, I'd often get caught staring out the windows at the parking lot. I'd shake on a smile when asked if everything was okay.

Nothing to see here.

The phone at work would ring with updates, threatening to expose the secrets of madness that were at home.

"Paolina, this is Dr. Gavino calling; how are you?" the grandmotherly voice of Viny's assigned psychiatrist wanted to know.

"Good, thank you." I whispered little else in response, lest any one of my teammates should hear.

She spoke in a clipped fashion: "Your sister, Viny. We had hoped she would calm down. But the medication is not working yet. Not as we would have liked."

Cocktail time!

This is worse than Mamma.

"What does that mean?" I asked, fearful of the answer to come.

"She's hearing voices," the doctor continued. "And seeing things. She's sad one minute. Over-happy the next. She keeps wandering. In and out of her room at night. And going into the hallways and other patients' rooms. Disturbing them."

I chuckled, inappropriately, imagining Viny visiting others at night—like the Tooth Fairy, only scarier. The visuals of the Polaroids Viny had asked Mamma to take of her just hours before I came home from my cruise flashed in my mind: She stood in front of our living room windows, wearing jeans and a blue-and-white-striped tank top. Her pudgy upper arms were pressed tightly against her body—her attempt, I assumed, to streamline her figure. Her skin glistened from sweat, her sunken eyes were underscored with dark, sleepless circles. And judging by the expression on her face, with her mouth half open, she was most likely screaming at Mamma to take the picture.

"She doesn't like to be alone," I mumbled into the receiver.

"Yes." Dr. Gavino paused. "Well, I'm scared for her and the other patients."

To hear the doctor share her fears for Viny when I had enough of my own wasn't helping.

"We put Viny in seclusion," she continued. "Increased the dosage to 5 milligrams of Stelazine. That should quiet the hallucinations. The lithium is a mood stabilizer. But I'm not seeing enough in her blood tests. Maybe we need more time, or to administer the drugs more often."

Jesus, they haven't a fucking clue.

A pinch of this. A dash of that.

I raised my eyes to the office ceiling, hoped that looking directly into the lights that hung overhead would stop my tears from falling. It was working. I inhaled more loudly than I had intended, then exhaled even louder.

"Paolina, I don't want you to worry," Dr. Gavino said, attempting to reassure me with words that never did. "This is all very normal."

Bullshit.

She promised to call with updates and let me know when we might discuss a discharge plan for Viny.

After hanging up the phone, it was business as usual. My mind kept wandering, especially when it shouldn't. Planning meetings, interviews, stories I would write—keeping on top of it all seemed futile.

Almost every night, before heading home to Mamma and before stopping by Papà's grave on the days I felt like doing that, I would spend an hour at The Women's Club. My weight seemed permanently set at 250 pounds, give or take 50 pounds. My exercise on the treadmill never went over thirty minutes, while my time in the whirlpool never dipped lower than thirty minutes. It was my time, and I was in charge of how I wanted to spend it. That meant entering the facility with a huge smile plastered on my face, and making some witty remark to Margie as I crossed in front of her office door on my way to the locker rooms.

"Hey, Paolina," Margie would call out to me. Then she'd resume her work. Sometimes she took the time to chat with me, as did the couple of members I had come to know when conducting the interviews for testimonial ads for the fitness center. But unless they initiated, I kept to myself.

WEEKS LATER, DR. GAVINO called for us to come get Viny.

I don't remember where my other siblings were—whether or not they joined me in picking her up or waited with Mamma at home, planning some sort of welcome home surprise. All I remember is on the day Viny came home, she was off-balance and disoriented from the drugs she'd been given. Her eyes rolled back in her head, her eyelids twitched nonstop. She complained that her neck was stiff.

Side effects of the drugs, they had said.

It was difficult to look at her, but what was worse was the grunge and the smell. I could barely get past it to help my sister.

"Vince, let's take a bath, okay?"

"No, I don't want to." Her response reminded me of a toddler's.

I steered my drugged-up sister to the bath. "Vince, it'll make you feel better. Promise."

I had her strip down naked and helped her into the tub.

"It's too hot."

"Okay, I'll add some cold. But we need the hot to get you clean."

Her body odor reminded me of Mamma's, and the amount of grease in her hair was so visible, it could have filled a bucket. I would have to wash it, too. And all I could think was how I would get myself clean after running my hands through her filth.

I conjured up my papà. There in the bathroom where he fell to his death. There in the same room where I watched him wash Mamma. She was naked in the tub, her enormous breasts sagging low, her entire back veiled by some yellow, smelly film of I don't know what. And my father was there with a sponge in his hands, on his knees, leaning over, washing her back.

Here was I. Same house. Same family. Same players. Same life.

I knelt in front of my sister. I took the sponge and soaked it in soap. And I washed every inch of her: her hair, her back, her privates.

And I hated every minute of it.

"Thank you, Pauley."

My sister's words only made it worse. I wished she were unaware. It would make things so much simpler. But regardless of how I truly felt inside, I had to pretend.

"You're welcome, Vince. Doesn't that feel better?"

I purposely made the water go into her ears and eyes. Something evil in me even thought about drowning her, ending the madness for us all.

What's wrong with you?

What would you do with Mamma?

Maybe you're the one who should be committed.

Viny tried to sound almost cheery. "Ya, thanks."

I dressed her in clean pajamas and put her to bed.

I retired myself, lowering my heavy body onto the thin mattress that still hailed from the bunk beds Viny and I had shared. In the silence, my mind raced. Plotted. Parts of me shuddered with fear. Parts of me ignited in rage. Parts of me caved in with shame. Inside, I splintered, with the exception of one unifying theme: I had to figure out how to get out of it. All of it.

I had had enough.

Whatever had been in me to survive up until that point had evaporated. Everything I had dreamt of doing or becoming no longer seemed even remotely possible. Worse still, I wasn't sure I even wanted it. What I was sure of was that I could no longer keep it together. I just wanted to sleep. Forever. I was too exhausted. While schizophrenia didn't seem to want to claim me, it didn't really have to. Madness had won. I conceded.

Well played.

SEATED IN THE WOMEN'S CLUB whirlpool, I found myself all alone. It was late, near closing time. The clock echoed in the cavernous room, and the gurgling froth of the bubbles seemed to keep in rhythm with it. I loved soaking in the spacious, warm waters of what felt like my own private tub. Why more women didn't use it, I would never know. But I was grateful they didn't.

Sinking down as far as I could, immersing my enormous body, letting the water lift it, I felt so weightless. It was the last feeling I wanted to feel before it all came to an end.

I had heard that if you let your gas stove seep, and then you came in and lit a match—KABOOM, you were a goner. That was the plan. That's what I wanted to be: gone. At twenty-eight, I had come to the conclusion that there was no other way out.

Calmly contemplating the final hours, the orchestrated ending to not only my life but that of Mamma and Viny, to whom I had become enslaved, I wondered if this was the peace Papà had felt on that night I had asked him if he was afraid to die.

Without hesitation, he'd said no. And now I felt the same way.

Mamma and Viny feared death, this much I knew. But they also feared life—at least, one that required you to be alone.

I already had tried once before to kill Mamma with that morning coffee twelve long years ago, but I had failed. Then again, I had not really planned it out that time.

This time would be different. It would be easy. A simple turn of a knob. A breathy blowout of the pilot light. A few moments to say some prayers. Or not. God didn't seem to be listening anyway.

And then it would be over. Quick and painless. That was important to me. Not for myself, but for Mamma and Viny. As much as I wanted them dead, I didn't want them to suffer.

I realized my mistake the last time was that I had left myself out of the equation—only wanting Mamma gone, with no thought of joining her. The resulting guilt, both over not having succeeded and, worse, over having been found out, had become a constant haunt. So this time, fair was fair: I would walk the talk and end my own life along with theirs. We would exit alone together.

Ironic, I know, to even wish someone dead, let alone a family member, and then to hatch plans to make it a reality, while in the same breath proclaiming your desire to protect them from suffering. It sounds crazy. Even to me. But that's what had become of my mind following a couple of decades of absorbing madness. No longer was I sure which one of us was more insane: the ones clinically diagnosed with mental illness or the one who took care of it all and was labeled "normal" by those who didn't know any better, the outsiders looking in.

All you wanted was to be normal.
Nothing to see here.

I was smart enough to keep my thoughts to myself. My years of practice that came with the seemingly genetic Sicilian code of keeping things inside the family had taught me to do that well. Sure, I had allowed internal wars of words to battle it out, crossing the synapses of my brain and causing me to think things that I assumed most normal people never would. Like thinking how my mother and sister had no clue what was coming their way tonight and at the same time thinking I had no clue how long I had been soaking—and almost giggling at those thoughts. But increasingly, I struggled to know what was right or wrong, appropriate or not. And it was becoming more and more difficult to stay silent and to not act on the things that popped into my mind.

I let myself slip even lower into the pool, the water warmly bubbling around me, a sort of greenish foam caressing parts of me I had made sure no one else would. Its sloshing and slurping bounced off the walls in the empty room. I inhaled, exaggerating my breathing. I could hear me, inside of me. In. Out. In. Out. The smell of chlorine stung the inside of my nose. Slowly, I blew the air out through my mouth as far as I could expel it, imagining my lungs shriveling up like a couple of wet plastic bags. And then I stopped. *So this is what it's like to no longer breathe*, I thought to myself. I barely held out ten seconds before my body rebelled.

I really didn't belong at the health club. I never had. I was there for one reason and one reason only: this oversize, jet-propelling tub. It was the one place I'd discovered that could make my morbidly obese body feel half its size and free enough to float.

Lost in my thoughts, I didn't hear Margie, the club's owner, approaching until she said, "Hey P, it's closing time. You been in here all night?"

I looked up at her. Margie was so kind. Her bright eyes seemed to change colors with her moods, like one of those rings.

"What time is it?" I asked.

"Eight o'clock. Everybody's gone home, except you and me. And I'm ready to go."

I just looked at her for the longest of moments. Then tears began to blur my vision. I leaned my head back, looking up at the lights, dunking my long brown curls, ready to blame any wayward tear on the water I'd been stewing in.

I stood up, shook it off. This was it. I was done. I was ready.

I lifted myself out of the water. How heavy I felt. How much I would miss that whirlpool.

Margie handed me a towel. I took hers and the one I had brought myself and wrapped both around me.

"You okay?" she asked.

I nodded, avoiding her gaze.

She put her hand on my forearm and turned me so she could look into my eyes. I'm not sure what she saw. I imagine that as a fitness professional, she would have seen a challenge: a mound of fat suffocating a five-foot-six frame; a block of Italian marble she would have loved—*I would have loved*—to chisel and set free, similar to Michelangelo's slaves. But she never seemed to notice. No one did. My fault. I never gave anybody any indication of what was going on inside my family, inside me.

Until this night, when I failed to keep the secrets hidden, and Margie saw something else—maybe a pair of big brown eyes, usually alert and engaged, now hollowed out and void.

She kept hold of my arm and put her other around my back, the whole while sort of steering me and moving me forward, as if I was physically impaired.

She softened the tone of her voice and nearly whispered to me, "You know, I want to talk to you about some more promotional stuff—since we're both here. You have a few minutes to come into my office?"

"It's late, Margie," I said.

"Just a couple of minutes, I promise," she said.

I promise. Just a couple of minutes. Neither ever turned out to be kept. And yet, even knowing this to be true, I couldn't seem to ever say or stick to "no."

Still wrapped in my towels, she led the way down the hall. All the other lights of the facility had been shut off, except for the one in her little office. Nothing much was in it: a desk, a phone, Margie, and me. She sat me down in one of the two chairs, while she stayed standing, hovering over me. I kept my head down, avoiding her gaze.

"You don't seem right to me tonight, Paolina. Everything okay?"

I hesitated for a moment. Everything okay? Everything. Okay. I let her words marinate in my mind. No. Nothing was okay.

I nodded. But I so wanted to tell her the truth. I needed to tell. Someone. Anyone. Not only to get it all off my chest, make my last confession, but to make sure someone knew. For a moment—just a split second, really—I thought it would be good for at least one person to know why I would torch my house, my mamma, my sister, myself.

I couldn't stand it if after it was over, no one had a clue why. Just as I couldn't stand it whenever I would hear or read on the news that someone had done what I was about to do or something similar, and so many people would shake their heads and wonder why or even say, "How could they? How crazy must they have been?"—or the opposite: "She seemed so normal." I hated it.

If there was one thing I had learned the hard way it was that crazy came in many forms, and it lurked within us all. While both my mamma and Viny were clinically diagnosed, my kind of crazy kept itself hidden. On the outside, I was fully functioning. On the inside, the secrets I was keeping were killing me. So while others shook their heads in disbelief or disapproval of the latest shooting or suicide or some other tragedy of the human spirit, I would always quietly nod and, deep down, fully understand why.

So, for just a moment, I wanted to tell Margie my plans and the reasoning behind them. Maybe then, people—especially my two other siblings, Caterina and Rosario—might understand afterward. Hell, they might even thank me.

But looking up into Margie's eyes, I changed my mind, instantaneously dismissed the thought. One look and I realized it wouldn't be fair to unload on her and for her, then, to carry the burden of having known, yet not been able to stop it. It was too much to go into. And besides, I just didn't have the time. I was on a mission to kill and be killed.

I tried to smile. "Everything's right as rain." I'd always liked that saying. Although I really had no clue what it meant. "Right as rain"? How was rain "right"? I mean, sure, I loved a wicked thunderstorm, but what was right about it? I wondered. And then I dismissed the thought, given that now I would never know.

Margie reached down and took my hand. "Sweetie, you seem a little 'off' tonight."

Now I was starting to get angry. I didn't need this. Not tonight. Not now. Not so late in the game. When a decision has been made, other points of view just aren't welcome. They only serve to cloud and confuse. And nothing ever changes. I had already accepted my fate. And I was too spent to entertain any alternatives that had the potential to change my plans.

"Margie, I'm fine. Really," I lied. "It's late. I still have to shower and change." I faked a laugh and tried to make my escape.

She wouldn't let me go. With one hand still holding on to me, she picked up the phone and started to dial. She kept her eyes locked on mine. "I have a friend. She's right around the corner. I want you to see her. Do that for me?"

Oh God, I thought. *Yet another someone who wants me to do something for them.*

"Margie, I wish I could, but—"

"Please, Paolina. Just this one last thing I'll ask of you."

I do not know what Margie saw in me that night. But I do know what I saw in her: fear. She was clearly afraid for me. Not of me. But for me. And I hated seeing that in her eyes and knowing it was because of me. She didn't deserve this. And I didn't need that guilt mounted onto the pile I already had amassed.

"Thirty minutes. That's all I have left to give."

I QUICKLY CHANGED BACK INTO my work clothes. Any thoughts of escaping left me when I found Margie waiting for me at the exit.

"I'll drive," she said.

"What about my car?" I asked as I followed to hers.

Margie offered only the hint of a smile in response.

Moments later, I slumped in the passenger seat of Margie's car as she drove the half-mile or so down the street and into the parking lot of a drab, single-story brick office complex. For the short duration of the trip, Margie babbled. I was silent, staring straight ahead, calculating in my mind the new timetable for what was to come. Now I needed to add time to get back to my car. I should have insisted on driving myself.

You should have.

Now you're stuck.

A life of obligation.

The voices were along for the ride. They seemed as tired as I was and just as ready for it to be over. Justifying the delay, I reasoned in my mind that this would be a good thing. After all, it wasn't even nine o'clock yet; there was still plenty of time before night's end. And the more I thought about it, the more I realized this might be a blessing in disguise, given the fact that the later I got home, the less chance there was that anyone else would still be awake.

We parked the car. Margie got out, came over to my side, and opened my door for me. I stepped out, avoiding her look of concern. Only one light glowed above one of the doors, just enough light to illuminate the sign to the left of it, which read, "Psychological Services." I can't be sure, but I think if I had seen that sign and been in the "right" state of mind, I would have run away. I did not need any further confirmation that as much as I tried to deny it, I, too, was crazy—that this apple had likely not fallen as far as she had thought from the family tree.

The door opened. A woman greeted us. She was petite and pixie-like; even her caramel-colored hair was cut in that cute pixie style. She looked like the girl next door. I wasn't sure of her age, but she was older than me and yet looked as if she had lived twenty years fewer than I had. She had such a warm smile, and eyes that sparkled. I felt welcomed from the moment I set eyes on her. Something inside of me wanted to be hugged by her. Even just to say good-bye.

"This is my friend Lynn," Margie said, passing me off to her. The pair nodded to one another, some secret between them exchanged. Margie left.

Lynn and I entered her office.

She led me through the perfectly clinical waiting room. Magazines galore, from *Psychology Today* to *Birds and Bloom* to *People*, littered the end tables. We moved past the empty receptionist desk and down the hall to Lynn's office. She let me step in first, and then closed the door behind me. First thing I noticed: she had lots of books. Second thing I noticed: I had never heard of a single one of them. Third thing I noticed: she had a couch—a soft, melted butter, come hither, hunter green leather couch. I plopped myself into it, let myself be swallowed up by it. I so wanted to lie down and go to sleep.

Lynn sat in a big leather captain's chair directly across from me, her yellow ruled pad of paper and pen at the ready.

"Margie says you're struggling," Her voice soothed, instantly making me feel safe. "What's going on?"

I tried to avoid eye contact. Even if I had wanted to talk to her, I didn't have time for a chat. And I still couldn't quite shake the thought that no one would understand why I needed to do what I had to do.

I stayed silent for a moment, then steeled my gaze and met Lynn's eyes. Calmly, confidently, I replied, "Nothing. Really."

Lynn looked at me. She was silent herself for a moment and then said the four little words that would begin to bring me back to life:

"Tell me about 'nothing.'"

EPILOGUE

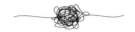

"This is the very worst wickedness:
That we refuse to acknowledge the passionate evil
that is in us. This makes us secret and rotten."
—D.H. Lawrence

I HAD TO PUT THE PAST behind me to finally move on. That truly began in earnest when I met Lynn, who would become my therapist for more than a decade. With her help, I would come to realize that "crazy" and "normal" were relative, and that both lived within each of us. I would understand that true insanity in life was to keep doing the same thing, always expecting different results. I would know the simple truth that each of us can change and save only ourselves, nobody else. And I would learn that it's okay to not be okay—that to fall apart and to get help were signs of strength, not weakness.

Words and beliefs would take on multi-layered meanings, "committed" being one:

1. Feeling dedication and loyalty to a cause, activity, or job; wholeheartedly dedicated—As in, *"She's committed to her role as a caregiver."*
2. To carry out or perpetrate (a mistake, crime, or immoral act)—As in, *"She committed such acts of desperation."*
3. Sending (someone) to be confined in a psychiatric hospital—As in, *"She had her mom and sister committed."*

No longer would I view life in black and white, fearing the gray.

Getting swallowed up by my circumstances had led me down some bunny holes that, had I not been introduced to Lynn on that fateful night, might have ended in a very tragic way. After a lifetime of serving as caregiver to crazy without question, I had joined the ranks of those whom society would say needed to be committed. The questions of *What is normal?* and *Who really can be called crazy?* were now joined by *How does being committed to a cause or a person or a belief have the potential to lead one to actually getting committed to a hospital?* There were no right and wrong answers for these questions and more that life asked of me and that I asked of myself. At least, not any I could find all on my own.

What was given to me—the roots of insanity in my family tree—was inescapable, but with Lynn's help, I sprouted the knowledge that every one of us is "crazy" or has the potential for becoming so. There will be times when we will align with what might be considered "normal," and times when we will fall outside of its accepted scope. Our passions and commitments may blur boundaries to the point where we may need to be committed, while those who would find themselves clinically diagnosed, labeled as insane, and actually committed may at times be the sanest among us.

The word or label of "crazy," I would conclude, was not the issue, any more so than "normal" or "committed" or any other word was for that matter; rather, the definitions we assigned to those words, the beliefs we had in them, and the stigmas we empowered were at fault. For at any given point during each individual's experiences in this world, the reality is that we ebb and flow along the spectrum of everything that makes us human. Our saving grace isn't in being perfect but in exposing our secrets, ending the shame that comes with them, and welcoming all parts as the sum of the whole.

What my story so far has taught me is that our true power is realized when we no longer fear the darkness, but embrace it. When we can see both sides as part of us and be at peace with both the light and the dark, we step into all of who we truly are.

Recognizing the madness that surrounds us and is within us and learning to channel it into magic, is how we defy gravity and unleash forces beyond what we can even imagine.

My own journey continues, embracing the madness laced with that spark of magic.

It is who I am, and I am exactly who I am meant to be.

PHOTO ALBUM

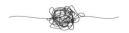

WHILE THE PAGES OF *COMMITTED* include letters and notes throughout to help tell the story, I want to also share some important images from my life.

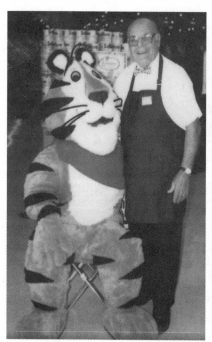

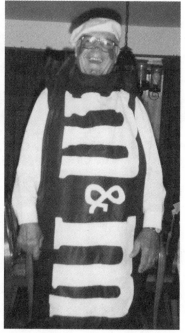

Papà with Tony the Tiger

Papà in his M&M Halloween costume

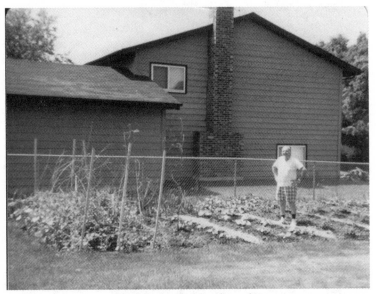

Papà in his beloved garden

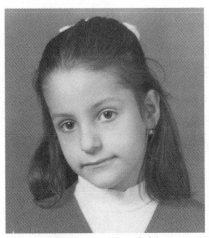

Viny as a shy child

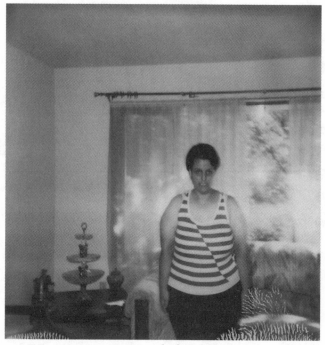

Viny in May 1992 just before being committed

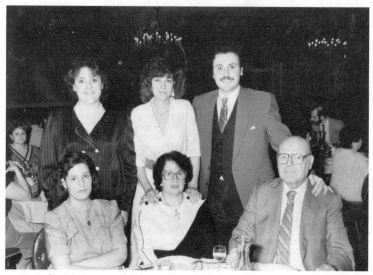

July 28, 1985—Milana family at an anniversary party

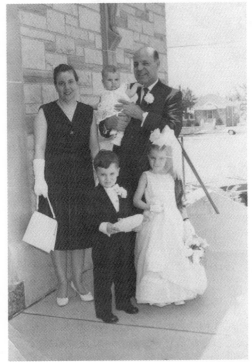

Milana family a few months after I was
born/two years before Viny's birth—Mamma
handmade my sister's flower girl dress

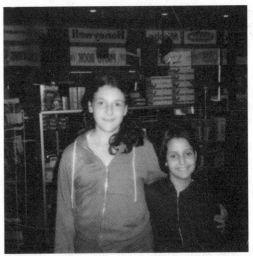

I'm with Crazy: A Love Story of Viny and Me

READING GROUP GUIDE

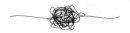

THE FOLLOWING QUESTIONS ABOUT *Committed* are intended as prompts to aid individual readers and book groups who may wish to discuss scenes, situations, and themes from this story. My hope is that this guide will help provide readers with a starting place from which to approach this book.

1. Why do you think the author has chosen *Committed* as her title? What significance does that word have in terms of mental illness and caregiving?
2. Every chapter is entitled with a word beginning with the letter C; why?
3. The concept of *normal* is one the author longs for. What do you consider to be normal, both in the story you just read and in your own life's story?
4. The word *crazy* sets off alarms for some of us. People may think the use of the word crazy is harmless; others believe giving negative value to the word contributes to marginalizing people. What's your opinion?
5. How would you have reacted to the situations detailed in this story? Would you have stayed to care for the people in your life? Have you? Or have you chosen not to?
6. Body image plays a role in Paolina's self-confidence. In what ways do the people in her life influence her perceptions of self?

7. What would you do differently if you were the author, trying to deal with her circumstances? What would you do the same? Why?

8. Consider Viny and her childhood loneliness, bullying, and learning disabilities. At what points might some intervention have put her on a different path?

9. When the author receives a check for just a bit more than the amount needed for her outstanding tuition at ISU, we might call that serendipity, just as seeing the license plate "LUV DAD" might be considered coincidence. Is it possible, however, that these and the other happenstances might be something other than random? If so, how might they be characterized?

10. When Papà dies, the family drifts further apart instead of closer together. Why do you think that happened? Have you ever experienced a death? Has it caused togetherness or separation?

11. How might it have felt for Mamma when she endured nights of Viny screaming at no one there, just as she had done years earlier? How do you think she might have felt realizing that she had passed mental illness on to her youngest daughter?

12. Consider the sibling relationships of Paolina's family, the ages and birth orders. How might those have factored into positions of being caregivers? In your own family, how are siblings alike and/or different? Why do you think that is so?

13. What are your thoughts about children who become caregivers or who take on adult roles in the absence of healthy parents? Do they suffer? Or are they better positioned to succeed as adults themselves as a result?

14. Why would the author end the story at the very point when she is planning a murder-suicide and seemingly by divine intervention meets a therapist who wants her to "tell me about 'nothing'"? Why would she leave the reader hanging?

15. "Tell me about 'nothing.'" As the author shared in the epilogue, this one line from the stranger who would become her therapist changed everything. What do you think about this line? What would "nothing" encompass from your own life?

16. Mental illness robs many people of any sense of control they might have formerly had in their lives. Thoughts can take on a life of their own and make us feel worthless or undeserving or as if something is wrong with us—whether we have a diagnosed disorder or not. Have your own thoughts ever spiraled out of control? If so, how did you manage?

17. Feeling trapped can lead to a sense of hopelessness and a lack of believing that one will ever be able to overcome their circumstances. Suffering in secret only worsens the situation. At what points would the people in this memoir have benefited from sharing what was going on in their minds and seeking the help they needed? Why do you think they chose to get through it on their own?

18. Paolina continuously sets her sights on giving just "one year" to things. Why do you think she does that? Is it a wise strategy or not wise at all?

19. Fear of judgment and the fear of consequences of allowing oneself to fall apart lead to pretending that everything is okay when it's not. The stigma associated with disclosing any kind of "not normal" or "crazy" thoughts and feelings often cause us to suffer in silence. How might knowing this help us and others be more open when we're not feeling okay?

20. Resilience is the capacity to recover quickly from difficulties. Some say it's the ability to constantly bounce back. In what ways do Paolina and others in this book exhibit resilience?

21. In the Epilogue, the author quotes D.H. Lawrence's words: "This is the very worst wickedness: That we refuse to acknowledge the passionate evil that is in us. This makes us secret and rotten." What do you think he meant by this?

ACKNOWLEDGMENTS

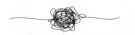

"Be bold and mighty forces shall come to your aid."
—JOHANN WOLFGANG VON GOETHE

THIS QUOTE HAS LONG BEEN one of my favorites, and I've lived my life trusting it and realizing its truth. Throughout my story, so many mighty forces—friends, family, colleagues, random run-ins, and circumstances—have influenced me and contributed to who I am today. Not wishing to accidentally leave anyone out, rather than name names, I simply wish to thank you all. I hope you know how much you mean to me. I am grateful for you being a part of my story, both the madness and the magic. I would not be who or what I am today without you.

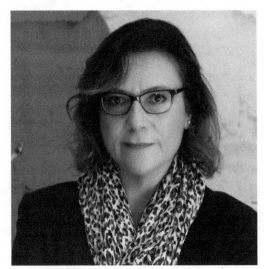

Author photo © Jennifer Carrillo

ABOUT THE AUTHOR

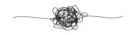

PUBLISHED AUTHOR, SPEAKER, PODCASTER, content producer, and Founder of Madness to Magic, Paolina Milana's mission is to share stories that celebrate the triumph of the human spirit and the power that lies within each of us to bring about change for the better. Her professional background includes telling other people's stories, both as a journalist and as a PR and digital media/marketing executive. She currently serves as a Court Appointed Special Advocate (CASA) for children in foster care as well as an empowering writing coach who uses storytelling to help people reimagine their lives, write their next chapters, and become the heroes of their own journeys. Paolina's first book, *The S Word* (She Writes Press, May 2015), earned the National Indie Excellence Award. *Seriously! Are We THERE Yet?!* (October 2020) is the first in her "children's book for adults" series, and *Miracle on Mall Drive* (November 2020) is her first novel. Her free podcast, *I'm with Crazy: A Love Story* is on Apple Podcasts. A proud first-generation Sicilian, Paolina is married and lives on the edge of the Angeles National Forest in Southern California. She welcomes readers to contact her at powerlina@madnesstomagic.com.

SELECTED TITLES FROM SHE WRITES PRESS

She Writes Press is an independent publishing company founded to serve women writers everywhere. Visit us at www.shewritespress.com.

At the Narrow Waist of the World: A Memoir by Marlena Maduro Baraf. $16.95, 978-1-63152-588-9. In this lush and vivid coming-of-age memoir about a mother's mental illness and the healing power of a loving Jewish and Hispanic extended family, young Marlena must pull away from her mother, leave her Panama home, and navigate the transition to an American world.

Implosion: Memoir of an Architect's Daughter by Elizabeth W. Garber. $16.95, 978-1-63152-351-9. When Elizabeth Garber, her architect father, and the rest of their family move into Woodie's modern masterpiece, a glass house, in 1966, they have no idea that over the next few years their family's life will be shattered—both by Woodie's madness and the turbulent 1970s.

The Coconut Latitudes: Secrets, Storms, and Survival in the Caribbean by Rita Gardner. $16.95, 978-1-63152-901-6. A haunting, lyrical memoir about a dysfunctional family's experiences in a reality far from the envisioned Eden—and the terrible cost of keeping secrets.

Raising Myself: A Memoir of Neglect, Shame, and Growing Up Too Soon by Beverly Engel. $16.95, 978-1-63152-367-0. A powerfully inspiring and unflinchingly honest story of how best-selling author and abuse recovery expert Beverly Engel made her way in the world—in spite of her mother's neglect and constant criticism, undergoing sexual abuse at nine, and being raped at twelve.

Patchwork: A Memoir of Love and Loss by Mary Jo Doig. $16.95, 978-1-63152-449-3. Part mystery and part inspirational memoir, *Patchwork* chronicles the riveting healing journey of one woman who, following the death of a relative, has a flashback that opens a dark passageway back to her childhood and the horrific secrets that have long been buried deep inside her psyche.

Baffled by Love: Stories of the Lasting Impact of Childhood Trauma Inflicted by Loved Ones by Laurie Kahn. $16.95, 978-1-63152-226-0. For three decades, Laurie Kahn has treated clients who were abused as children—people who were injured by someone who professed to love them. Here, she shares stories from her own rocky childhood along with those of her clients, weaving a textured tale of the all-too-human search for the "good kind of love."